INFLAMMATION TO TRANSFORMATION:

The ultimate Science-Based Eat, Heal and full Body Transformation in one Week

BY

Dr. Klein Houghton

Copyright © by Dr. Klein Houghton 2024.

All rights reserved.

Table of Contents

INTRODUCTION

Welcome to Your Transformation Process!

Welcome to "Inflammation to Transformation: A definitive Science-Based Eat, Mend, and Full Body Transformation in 1-Week." If you're holding this book, you're probably looking for a significant Transformation in your well-being and prosperity. You may be battling with tenacious exhaustion, gut-related issues, weight gain, or persistent Inflammation. Maybe you've attempted various weight control plans and health programs, just to wind up back where you began, baffled and discouraged.

This book is intended to offer you a new beginning, an experimentally supported, comprehensive way to deal with recuperating your body from the back to front. Throughout the following seven days, you'll leave on a groundbreaking excursion that won't just assist you with shedding undesirable pounds yet in addition decrease Inflammation, recuperate your gut, and reestablish your energy and essentialness.

The Science behind Inflammation and Weight Management

Inflammation is a characteristic reaction of the safe framework to injury or contamination. In any case, when Inflammations becomes persistent, it can prompt a large group of medical conditions, including weight gain, gut-related issues, and, surprisingly, constant illnesses like diabetes and coronary illness. Persistent Inflammation can upset your body's hormonal equilibrium, disable supplement ingestion, and debilitate your resistant framework. Understanding the science behind aggravation is significant to resolving these issues at their underlying driver.

Ongoing examinations have shown areas of strength between constant Inflammation and weight. At the point when your body is in a condition of persistent Inflammation, it clutches fat as a defensive component. This makes it challenging to get in shape as well as makes way for additional unexpected issues. By tending to aggravation straightforwardly, you can break this cycle and make ready for economical weight reduction and work on generally speaking wellbeing.

How This 7-Day Plan Functions

This book presents a far-reaching, science-based plan to assist you with changing your body and well-being in only multiple weeks. The arrangement is separated into three primary parts: eating, mending, and changing.

1. Eating: The food varieties you eat assume a pivotal part in either advancing or decreasing Inflammation. This plan accentuates mitigating food varieties plentiful in cancer prevention agents, nutrients, and minerals. You'll figure out how to get ready heavenly, supplement thick dinners that help your body's recuperating processes and advance weight reduction.

2. Healing: Recuperating your gut is a basic part of this arrangement. The gut is home to trillions of microorganisms that impact everything from absorption to resistance capability. A sound gut microbiome is fundamental for lessening Inflammation and supporting by and large well-being. This plan incorporates probiotics, prebiotics, and other gut-mending food varieties to reestablish harmony in your gut-related framework.

3. Transforming: Genuine Transformation requires a comprehensive methodology that incorporates active work and care rehearses. This plan consolidates delicate yet successful activities that help digestion and lessen pressure. Also, care methods, for example, contemplation and profound breathing activities are incorporated to assist you with overseeing pressure and backing mental prosperity.

Putting forth Practical Objectives

Before jumping into the arrangement, putting forth sensible and reachable goals is significant. While the essential focal point of this book is to assist you with accomplishing a critical Transformation in a multi-week, it's likewise about establishing the groundwork for long-haul well-being and health. Think about your ongoing well-being status, recognize explicit regions you might want to improve, and set clear, quantifiable objectives. Keep in mind, that is an excursion, and each step you take carries you nearer to your definitive well-being and health objectives.

Fundamental Apparatuses and Fixings

To prevail in this 7-day plan, you'll have to set up a couple of fundamental devices and fixings. These incorporate essential kitchen gear like a blender, food processor, and quality cookware. Stock up on new, entire food sources like natural products, vegetables, lean proteins, nuts, seeds, and matured food varieties. Furthermore, consider consolidating excellent enhancements like omega-3 unsaturated fats and probiotics to help your body's recuperating processes.

Pre-Transformation Detox Tips

Before beginning the 7-day plan, it's painful to go through a delicate detox to set up your body for Transformation. This includes killing handled food varieties, sugar, caffeine, and liquor from your eating routine. All things being equal, centers around hydrating with a lot of water, natural teas, and green juices. This pre-Transformation detox will assist with resetting your body, diminish aggravation, and advance supplement ingestion.

Step by step Breakdown

The center of this book is the step-by-step plan intended to direct you through your Transformation process. Every day incorporates:

- **Feast Plans:** Painstakingly created dinner plans highlighting mitigating, gut-recuperating food varieties. Every recipe is intended to be both delectable and supplement thick, making it simple to stay on track.
- **Practice Routines:** Delicate yet compelling activities that help digestion, further develop the course, and lessen pressure. These schedules are appropriate for all wellness levels and should be possible at home with insignificant gear.
- **Care Practices:** Everyday care practices to assist you with overseeing pressure, further developing concentration, and backing mental prosperity. These incorporate strategies like contemplation, profound breathing activities, and journaling.

I.   Launching Your Transformation

Day 1 is tied in with launching your Transformation. You'll start with a supplement-stuffed calming smoothie for breakfast, trailed by a gut-recuperating salad for lunch and a lean protein with veggies for supper. The delicate yoga routine will assist with further developing adaptability and decreasing pressure, while profound breathing activities will uphold unwinding and care.

II.   Supporting Your Digestion

On Day 2, it centers on the movements to support your digestion. You'll partake in an omega-3-rich breakfast bowl, a matured food variety feast for lunch, and a calming soup for supper. The cardio meeting will get your heart siphoning and assist with consuming calories, while the directed reflection will advance unwinding and mental clearness.

III.   Recuperating Your Gut

Day 3 is committed to mending your gut. Probiotic-rich yogurt parfaits, entire grain wraps, and fish and veggie pan-fried food are on the menu. Strength-preparing activities will assist with building muscle and lifting digestion, while journaling will give an outlet to reflect and stress the board.

IV.   Decreasing Aggravation

On Day 4, you'll zero in on decreasing Inflammation with turmeric and ginger tea breakfast, a calming power bowl for lunch and a quinoa and veggie skillet for supper. Pilate's activities will reinforce your center and further develop adaptability, while perception methods will uphold mental prosperity

V. Upgrading Supplement Retention

Day 5 is tied in with upgrading supplement retention. You'll begin with a green smoothie, appreciate lentil soup for lunch, and heat chicken with simmered vegetables for supper. Extreme cardio exercise (HIIT) will support your digestion and consume fat, while an appreciation practice will cultivate a positive outlook.

VI. Improving Gut Wellbeing

On Day 6, you'll improve gut well-being with chia seed pudding for breakfast, avocado and bean salad for lunch, and shrimp and veggie pan sear for supper. A tomfoolery dance exercise will keep you moving and inspire your spirits, while moderate muscle unwinding will help you loosen up and lessen strain.

VII. Accomplishing Full-Body Transformation

Day 7 denotes the zenith of your Transformation process. You'll partake in a berry and nut smoothie for breakfast, a rainbow veggie bowl for lunch and lean meat with steamed vegetables for supper. A full-body extending routine will upgrade adaptability and unwinding, while reflection and preparation will make way for keeping up with your advancement.

Supporting Your Transformation

After finishing the 7-day plan, supporting your transformation is fundamental. This part gives direction on long-haul dinner arranging, integrating exercise into your everyday schedule, and proceeding with care rehearses. You'll likewise track down ways to explore normal difficulties and keep up with inspiration.

Normal Difficulties and Arrangements

Setting out on an extraordinary excursion isn't without its difficulties. This part tends to normal hindrances like desires, time imperatives, and social circumstances. You'll track down functional arrangements and procedures to remain focused and defeat any obstacles that come in your direction.

Genuine Transformations

Nothing is more moving than catching wind of genuine Transformations. This part includes tributes and examples of overcoming adversity from people who have finished the 7-day plan. Their encounters and experiences will propel and urge you to remain focused on your excursion.

Supplements and Extra Assets

The reference sections incorporate various extra assets to help your Transformation. You'll track down definite recipes, shopping records, and further understanding proposals. These assets are intended to make your process as smooth and agreeable as could be expected.

References and Logical Investigations

This book is grounded in logical examination and proof-based rehearses. The references segment gives a far-reaching rundown of the examinations and sources that help the standards and procedures illustrated in the arrangement. This straightforwardness guarantees you can trust the data and feel positive about your excursion.

Affirmations and Emotionally supportive networks

In conclusion, the affirmations area perceives the people and emotionally supportive networks that have added to the production of this book. From medical services experts and scientists to loved ones, this excursion wouldn't be imaginable without their help and mastery.

Your Transformation Starts Now

As you set out on this excursion, recollect that Transformation is an interaction that requires responsibility, persistence, and self-sympathy. This book is your aide and buddy, furnishing you with the device's information, and backing you want to accomplish a better, more joyful you.

Take a full breath, open your psyche, and prepare to Transformation your life. Your excursion from Inflammation to Transformation begins now. How about we begin!

CHAPTER 1: Figuring out Inflammation

1.11 What is Inflammation?

Inflammation is a natural reaction of body tissues to hurtful upgrades, like microbes, harmed cells, or aggravations. It is a defensive instrument intended to kill the underlying reason for cell injury, get out necrotic cells and tissues harmed from the first affront, and start tissue fix. Aggravation can be sorted into two kinds: intense and persistent, each with particular attributes and suggestions for well-being.

Intense Inflammation

Intense Inflammation is the body's quick reaction to injury or contamination. It is portrayed by the fast beginning of side effects like redness, heat, expansion, agony, and loss of capability. This sort of Inflammation is fundamental for endurance, as it assists the body with warding off diseases and recuperating wounds. For instance, if you cut your finger, the region around the cut will become excited as your body's safe framework sends white platelets and different substances to the site to battle any attacking microbes and begin the mending system.

The course of intense aggravation includes a few stages:

1. Recognition of the Harmful Agent: The body identifies unsafe boosts, like microbes or harmed cells, through design acknowledgment receptors (PRRs) on invulnerable cells.

2. Recruitment of Invulnerable Cells: Incendiary arbiters, like cytokines and chemokines, are delivered, which draw in safe cells like neutrophils and macrophages to the site of injury.

3. Removal of the Agent: Invulnerable cells work to wipe out the hurtful improvements through processes like phagocytosis, where they overwhelm and process microbes or trash.

4. Resolution of Inflammation: When the hurtful improvements are eliminated, the Inflammation dies down, and the tissue starts to fix itself. Calming signals help to determine the Inflammation and reestablish typical tissue capability.

Intense Inflammation is commonly fleeting, enduring from a couple of hours to a couple of days, and is settled once the unsafe boosts are disposed of, and the mending system is in progress.

Persistent Aggravation

Persistent Inflammation, then again, is a drawn-out and frequently poor-quality provocative reaction that continues for weeks, months, or even years. Dissimilar to intense Inflammation, which is a valuable and fundamental piece of the recuperating system, persistent Inflammation can impede well-being. It can happen when the body neglects to dispose of the reason for intense aggravation when there is an immune system reaction where the body goes after its tissues or because of nonstop openness to aggravations.

A few variables can add to constant Inflammation, including:

- **Diligent Infections:** Diseases that are not enough cleared by the resistant framework can prompt continuous aggravation. For instance, constant diseases with microscopic organisms like Helicobacter pylori can cause long-haul Inflammation in the gut lining, prompting conditions like gastritis and peptic ulcers.

- **Immune system Disorders:** In immune system sicknesses, the resistant framework erroneously goes after the body's tissues, causing persistent Inflammation. Models incorporate rheumatoid joint pain, where the invulnerable framework focuses on the joints, and lupus, which can influence numerous organs.

- **Drawn out Openness to Irritants:** Nonstop openness to hurtful substances like tobacco smoke, contamination, or modern synthetic compounds can cause constant aggravation in different tissues. For example, smoking can prompt ongoing Inflammation in the lungs, adding to sicknesses like constant obstructive aspiratory illness (COPD) and cellular breakdown in the lungs.

- **Way of life Factors**: Terrible eating routine, absence of activity, ongoing pressure, and deficient rest can all add to a condition of constant poor-quality Inflammation. Counts calories high in sugar, refined starches, and unfortunate fats can advance Inflammation, while customary active work and stress the executive's methods can assist with decreasing it.

The Job of Aggravation in Wellbeing and Illness

While Inflammation is a characteristic and fundamental piece of the body's protection system, persistent Inflammation can prompt different medical problems. Understanding the double idea of aggravation is pivotal for perceiving its effect on our well-being.

The Advantageous Job of Aggravation

Intense aggravation is essential for mending and assurance against diseases. It assists the body with warding off microbes, fixing harmed tissues, and re-establishing homeostasis. Without

Inflammation, even minor wounds or contaminations could become dangerous, as the body would not be able to guard itself.

For instance, during bacterial contamination, Inflammation detaches and obliterates the attacking microbes. White platelets, especially neutrophils, are selected to the disease site, where they immerse and kill the microorganisms. This cycle disposes of the disease as well as forestalls its spread to different pieces of the body.

Additionally, on account of tissue injury, Inflammation assists start the maintenance with handling. At the point when you sprain your lower leg, the incendiary reaction helps eliminate harmed cells and tissues, advances the arrangement of fresh blood vessels, and works with the maintenance of the harmed tissue. This interaction is fundamental for reestablishing capability and forestalling further harm.

The Inconvenient Job of Constant Aggravation

While intense aggravation is useful, constant Inflammation can have extreme ramifications for well-being. Drawn-out Inflammation can harm sound tissues and organs, prompting a scope of persistent illnesses. The absolute most normal circumstances related to persistent Inflammation include:

1. Cardiovascular Disease: Persistent Inflammation is a critical gamble factor for cardiovascular sicknesses, for example, atherosclerosis, coronary episodes, and strokes. Aggravation adds to the arrangement of plaques in the conduits, which can burst and cause blood clumps, prompting coronary failures or strokes.

2. Type 2 Diabetes: Inflammation assumes a critical part in the improvement of insulin opposition, a sign of type 2 diabetes. Incendiary cytokines can obstruct insulin flagging, making it challenging for the body to manage glucose levels.

3. Obesity: Ongoing aggravation is in many cases seen in people with stoutness. Fat tissue (muscle to fat ratio) can deliver provocative cytokines, which add to metabolic brokenness and increment the gamble of weight-related infections like sort 2 diabetes, cardiovascular illness, and certain malignant growths.

4. Autoimmune Diseases: Persistent Inflammation is a critical component of immune system sicknesses like rheumatoid joint pain, lupus, and various sclerosis. In these circumstances, the safe framework assaults solid tissues, causing Inflammation and harm to joints, skin, and different organs.

5. Cancer: Constant aggravation is connected to the turn of events and movement of particular kinds of malignant growth. Incendiary cells and arbiters can advance cancer development, intrusion, and metastasis. For instance, ongoing Inflammation in the colon, as found in conditions like ulcerative colitis, builds the gamble of colorectal malignant growth.

6. Neurodegenerative Diseases: Inflammation is progressively perceived as a contributing variable in neurodegenerative sicknesses like Alzheimer's and Parkinson's illness. Constant aggravation in the mind can prompt the collection of harmful proteins and neuronal harm, disabling mental capability and adding to sickness movement.

The Sub-atomic and Cell Premise of Aggravation

To comprehend Inflammation completely, it's fundamental to dive into the atomic and cell components that support this intricate cycle. Inflammation includes an organized reaction of different insusceptible cells, flagging particles, and fiery middle people.

Vital participants in Aggravation

1. Immune Cells: A few kinds of resistant cells assume basic parts in Inflammation, including:

 - **Neutrophils**: These are the specialists on call for contamination or injury. They are profoundly powerful at overwhelming and obliterating microbes through a cycle called phagocytosis.

 - **Macrophages:** These cells are engaged with both the inception and goal of Inflammation. They can inundate microbes and trash, emit provocative middle people, and advance tissue fixes.

 - **Lymphocytes:** These incorporate Immune system microorganisms and B cells, which are critical for versatile resistance. Lymphocytes can assist with directing the invulnerable reaction, while B cells produce antibodies to kill microbes.

 - **Pole Cells:** These cells discharge receptors and other incendiary arbiters that add to the beginning phases of aggravation, for example, expanded blood-stream and vascular penetrability.

2. **Inflammatory Mediators**: Different atoms intervene in provocative reaction, including:

a. **Cytokines:** These are flagging proteins delivered by resistant cells that control Inflammation. Models incorporate interleukins (ILs), cancer putrefaction factor (TNF), and interferons (IFNs).

b. **Chemokines:** These are a subset of cytokines that explicitly draw in safe cells to the site of Inflammation. They assume a critical part in enlisting neutrophils, macrophages, and different cells to the impacted region.

c. **Prostaglandins:** These lipid compounds are created at the site of aggravation and add to the agony, fever, and enlarging. They are engaged with vasodilation and expanding vascular penetrability.

d. **Histamine:** Delivered by pole cells, receptors make veins expand and turn out to be more penetrable, permitting invulnerable cells to effortlessly arrive at the site of Inflammation more.

3. **Signaling Pathways:** Fiery flagging pathways are enacted in light of destructive improvements. These pathways include:

- **Atomic Component kappa B (NF-κB):** NF-κB is a record factor that controls the outflow of numerous provocative qualities. It is enacted by different provocative upgrades and assumes a focal part in organizing the resistant reaction.
- **Mitogen-Enacted Protein Kinases (MAPKs):** These kinases are associated with sending signals from the phone surface to the core, prompting the development of fiery go-betweens.

1.12 Acute versus chronic Inflammation

Aggravation is the body's defensive reaction to injury, disease, or hurtful boosts. While aggravation is significant for recuperating and protection, it can appear in Transformation structures with shifting ramifications for well-being. Aggravation is extensively classified into two kinds: intense and ongoing. Each type has particular attributes, components, and impacts on the body. Understanding the distinctions between intense and constant aggravation is fundamental for perceiving their jobs in well-being and illness.

Acute Inflammation

Intense Inflammation is the body's quick and momentary reaction to injury or disease. It is a basic piece of the body's guard system and is fundamental for mending and recuperation. The trademark indications of intense Inflammation are redness, heat, enlarging, agony, and loss of capability. These side effects result from the perplexing interaction of cell and sub-atomic occasions that happen at the site of injury or disease.

The Course of Acute Inflammation

The intense provocative reaction can be separated into a few phases:

1. Recognition of Destructive Stimuli: The body's resistant framework perceives unsafe upgrades like microbes (microorganisms, infections, and parasites), harmed cells, or aggravations through design acknowledgment receptors (PRRs) on insusceptible cells. These receptors identify microorganism-related atomic examples (PAMPs) and harm-related sub-atomic examples (DAMPs).

2. Release of Provocative: Endless supply of destructive boosts, insusceptible cells, for example, macrophages and pole cells discharge different fiery go-betweens, including cytokines, chemokines, receptors, and prostaglandins. These go-betweens start and direct the fiery reaction.

3. Vasodilatation and Expanded Permeability: Incendiary middle people make veins enlarge (vasodilation) and become more penetrable. This permits insusceptible cells, liquid, and proteins to leave the circulation system and enter the impacted tissue. The expanded bloodstream brings about redness and intensity, while the aggregation of liquid causes enlarging.

4. Recruitment of Safe Cells: Chemokines draw in resistant cells, like neutrophils and monocytes, to the site of Inflammation. Neutrophils are among the people on call and assume a vital part in phagocytosing (immersing and processing) microbes and garbage. Monocytes separate into macrophages, which proceed with the course of phagocytosis and assist with arranging the invulnerable reaction.

5. **Elimination of Destructive Stimuli**: Resistant cells work to dispose of the unsafe boosts through cycles like phagocytosis and the arrival of antimicrobial substances. This helps clear the contamination or eliminate harmed tissue.

6. Resolution of Inflammation: When the hurtful improvements are disposed of, the body starts calming cycles to determine the Inflammation and advance tissue fix. Calming cytokines and development factors assist with reestablishing typical tissue capability and forestalling exorbitant harm.

Results of Acute Inflammation

Intense Inflammation regularly settles within a couple of hours to a couple of days, contingent upon the seriousness of the injury or disease. The essential results of intense Inflammation include:

- o **Complete Resolution:** Generally speaking, intense Inflammation prompts the total disposal of the hurtful improvements and full recuperation of the impacted tissue. This is the best result and implies effective mending.
- o **Boil Formation:** Assuming that the contamination is serious or challenging to dispense with, a sore might shape. A sore is a restricted assortment of discharge (dead neutrophils, tissue cells, and microbes) that is walled off by the body to forestall the spread of disease. Abscesses might require clinical mediation to deplete and treat.
- o **Constant Inflammation**: If the intense fiery reaction isn't adequate to dispense with the unsafe improvements or on the other hand assuming the provocative signs endure, intense aggravation can Transformation into persistent Inflammation. This delayed reaction can prompt tissue harm and long-haul medical problems.

Chronic Inflammation

Chronic Inflammation is a drawn-out and frequently second-rate provocative reaction that endures for weeks, months, or even years. Dissimilar to intense Inflammation, which is a quick and self-restricting reaction, constant Inflammation is described by the persistent presence of provocative middle people and resistant cells. Persistent Inflammation can happen when the body neglects to dispense with the reason for intense aggravation when there is an immune system reaction, or because of continuous openness to aggravations.

Reasons for chronic Inflammation

A few elements can add to the improvement of persistent Inflammation:

1. Persistent Infections: Contaminations that are not satisfactorily cleared by the resistant framework can prompt continuous Inflammation. For instance, ongoing contaminations with microorganisms like Helicobacter pylori can cause long-haul Inflammation in the gut lining, prompting conditions like gastritis and peptic ulcers.

2. Autoimmune Disorders: In immune system illnesses, the resistant framework erroneously goes after the body's tissues, causing persistent Inflammation. Models incorporate rheumatoid joint inflammation, where the resistant framework focuses on the joints, and lupus, which can influence numerous organs.

3. Prolonged Openness to Irritants: Constant openness to destructive substances like tobacco smoke, contamination, or modern synthetic compounds can cause ongoing aggravation in different tissues. For example, smoking can prompt persistent Inflammation in the lungs, adding to sicknesses like constant obstructive pneumonic illness (COPD) and cellular breakdown in the lungs.

4. Lifestyle Factors: Terrible eating routine, absence of activity, constant pressure, and inadequate rest can all add to a condition of ongoing second-rate Inflammation. Abstains from food high in sugar, refined carbs, and undesirable fats can advance Inflammation, while normal active work and stress the executive's procedures can assist with diminishing it.

Instruments of chronic Inflammation

Constant Inflammation includes a complicated retransformation of insusceptible cells, provocative go-betweens, and flagging pathways. Key elements of persistent Inflammation include:

> **Tenacious Presence of Invulnerable Cells**: Constant Inflammation is described by the continuous enrollment and initiation of safe cells like macrophages, lymphocytes, and plasma cells. These cells discharge provocative middle people that sustain the incendiary reaction.

> **Tissue Harm and Repair:** Constant aggravation can prompt patterns of tissue harm and fix. Fiery go-betweens can cause cell harm, while the body endeavors to fix the tissue through fibrosis (arrangement of scar tissue). Over the long haul, this can bring about the deficiency of typical tissue capability and the improvement of ongoing sicknesses.

> **Favorable to Fiery Cytokines:** Ongoing aggravation is related to the persistent creation of supportive of provocative cytokines, for example, growth corruption factor (TNF), interleukin-6 (IL-6), and interleukin-1 (IL-1). These cytokines assume a focal part in supporting the provocative reaction and advancing tissue harm.

> **Oxidative Stress:** Ongoing aggravation is many times joined by oxidative pressure, which happens when there is lopsidedness between the creation of responsive oxygen species (ROS) and the body's cell reinforcement guards. ROS can harm cell parts like DNA, proteins, and lipids, further compounding Inflammation and tissue harm.

Wellbeing Ramifications of Chronic Inflammation

Constant Inflammation is a significant supporter of the turn of events and movement of various persistent illnesses. Understanding the well-being ramifications of constant Inflammation is urgent for perceiving its effect on general well-being and prosperity.

1. **Cardiovascular Disease:** Ongoing Inflammation is a huge gamble factor for cardiovascular infections, for example, atherosclerosis, coronary episodes, and strokes. Aggravation adds to the arrangement of plaques in the courses, which can crack and cause blood clusters, prompting coronary failures or strokes.

2. **Type 2 Diabetes:** Inflammation assumes a critical part in the improvement of insulin obstruction, a sign of type 2 diabetes. Incendiary cytokines can impede insulin flagging, making it hard for the body to direct glucose levels.

3. **Obesity:** Persistent aggravation is in many cases seen in people with corpulence. Fat tissue (muscle versus fat) can deliver fiery cytokines, which add to metabolic brokenness and increment the gamble of heftiness-related illnesses like sort 2 diabetes, cardiovascular sickness, and certain malignant growths.

4. **Autoimmune Diseases:** Persistent Inflammation is a vital element of immune system illnesses like rheumatoid joint inflammation, lupus, and numerous sclerosis. In these circumstances, the resistant framework assaults sound tissues, causing aggravation and harming joints, skin, and different organs.

5. **Cancer:** Persistent aggravation is connected to the turn of events and movement of particular sorts of malignant growth.

Fiery cells and go-betweens can advance cancer development, attack, and metastasis. For instance, ongoing Inflammation in the colon, as found in conditions like ulcerative colitis, builds the gamble of colorectal malignant growth.

6. Neurodegenerative Diseases: Inflammation is progressively perceived as a contributing element in neurodegenerative sicknesses like Alzheimer's and Parkinson's illness. Ongoing Inflammation in the cerebrum can prompt the gathering of poisonous proteins and neuronal harm, hindering mental capability and adding to illness movement.

Overseeing and decreasing chronic inflammation

Given the huge effect of constant aggravation on well-being, it is fundamental to embrace methodologies to oversee and lessen Inflammation. Here are a few viable methodologies:

1. Healthy Diet: Embracing a calming diet rich in natural products, vegetables, entire grains, lean proteins, and sound fats can assist with lessening Inflammation. Food varieties high in cancer prevention agents, omega-3 unsaturated fats, and fiber are especially advantageous.

2. Regular Exercise: Participating in ordinary actual work can assist with diminishing Inflammation and work on by and large wellbeing. Go for the gold 150 minutes of moderate-power practice or 75 minutes of energetic power practice each week.

3. Stress Management: Constant pressure can add to Inflammation. Practice pressure-decreasing strategies like reflection, profound breathing activities, yoga, and care to oversee feelings of anxiety.

4. Adequate Sleep: Guarantee you get sufficient helpful rest every evening. Go for the gold long stretches of value rest to help generally speaking well-being and decrease Inflammation.

5. Avoiding Smoking and Restricting Alcohol: Try not to smoke and restrict liquor utilization, as both can add to persistent Inflammation.

1.13 The Job of Inflammation in Medical Problems

Inflammation is an indispensable natural reaction to hurtful boosts, like microorganisms, harmed cells, or aggravations. It assumes an essential part in the body's protection and mending processes. In any case, when Inflammation becomes ongoing, it can add to a wide exhibit of medical problems. Understanding what Inflammation works and what it means for different frameworks in the body is fundamental for overseeing and forestalling these circumstances.

The Double Idea of inflammation

Inflammation can be both a companion and an enemy. Intense aggravation is valuable and important for endurance. It assists the body with battling contaminations, recuperating wounds, and answering wounds. Nonetheless, when Inflammation perseveres over a significant stretch, it becomes ongoing and can prompt various medical issues. Constant Inflammation is a quiet and tricky condition that frequently slips through the cracks until it causes critical harm.

1. Intense Inflammation: The Body's Quick Response

Intense Inflammation is the body's quick reaction to injury or contamination. It is portrayed by the exemplary indications of redness, heat, expansion, agony, and loss of capability. These side effects result from the expanded bloodstream, insusceptible cell movement, and the arrival of provocative middle people at the site of injury or contamination.

2. Persistent Inflammation: The Drawn-out Response

Persistent Inflammation, then again, is a drawn-out and frequently poor-quality fiery reaction that can keep going for quite a long time or even years. It can result from tireless diseases, continuous openness to unsafe substances, immune system responses, or way of life factors like less than stellar eating routine, absence of activity, and stress. Persistent Inflammation is a huge supporter of the improvement of numerous ongoing illnesses.

a.   Cardiovascular Illnesses

Quite possibly the most deeply grounded association between ongoing Inflammation and illness is in cardiovascular well-being. Persistent Inflammation assumes a basic part in the turn of events and movement of atherosclerosis, the development of greasy stores (plaques) in the walls of supply routes. These plaques can confine blood stream and, on the off chance that they burst, can prompt coronary episodes or strokes.

b. Atherosclerosis and Inflammation

Atherosclerosis starts with harm to the endothelium, the inward coating of veins. This harm can be brought about by elements, for example, hypertension, elevated cholesterol, smoking, and constant Inflammation. At the point when the endothelium is harmed, it sets off an incendiary reaction. White platelets, principally macrophages, are drawn to the site and start to overwhelm cholesterol particles, framing greasy streaks.

Over the long run, these greasy streaks form into bigger plaques. Constant Inflammation propagates this interaction by proceeding to enroll safe cells and advancing the development of the plaques. The provocative middle people can likewise debilitate the stringy cap that covers the plaques, making them bound to burst. A cracked plaque can prompt the development of blood coagulation, which can impede the bloodstream and cause respiratory failure or stroke.

c. C-Receptive Protein (CRP) and Cardiovascular Risk

C-receptive protein (CRP) is a marker of Inflammation that is ordinarily estimated in blood tests. Raised degrees of CRP are related to an expanded gamble of cardiovascular illnesses. CRP is delivered by the liver in light of provocative signs, and undeniable levels show that there is continuous Inflammation in the body. Checking CRP levels can assist with evaluating the gamble of cardiovascular occasions and guide preventive measures.

d. Metabolic Problems and Diabetes

Persistent Inflammation is likewise a critical figure in the improvement of metabolic problems, including type 2 diabetes and weight. These circumstances are frequently interrelated and can make an endless loop of Inflammation and metabolic brokenness.

e. **Stoutness and Inflammation**

Fat tissue, or muscle versus fat, isn't simply a capacity terminal for overabundance of energy. Additionally, a functioning endocrine organ produces chemicals and fiery middle people. In people with corpulence, fat tissue becomes amplified and broken, prompting the expanded creation of favorable to fiery cytokines, for example, growth corruption factor-alpha (TNF-α) and interleukin-6 (IL-6).

These provocative cytokines add to insulin obstruction, a condition where the body's cells become less receptive to insulin. Insulin obstruction is a significant gamble factor for type 2 diabetes. The ongoing second-rate Inflammation related to stoutness propagates the pattern of metabolic brokenness, making it challenging to accomplish and keep a solid weight.

f. **Type 2 Diabetes and Inflammation**

In type 2 diabetes, persistent Inflammation worsens insulin opposition and beta-cell brokenness. Beta cells in the pancreas produce insulin, and their hindrance is a sign of diabetes. Fiery arbiters can straightforwardly harm beta cells, decreasing their capacity to deliver insulin. In addition, aggravation obstructs insulin-flagging pathways, making it harder for the body to direct blood glucose levels.

Tending to constant aggravation through way of life Transformations, for example, embracing a calming diet and participating in ordinary active work, can further develop insulin awareness and assist with overseeing type 2 diabetes.

g. **Immune system Sicknesses**

Immune system sicknesses are conditions where the insusceptible framework erroneously goes after the body's tissues, prompting constant aggravation and tissue harm. There are more than 80 different immune system infections, including rheumatoid joint pain, lupus, various sclerosis, and provocative gut illness (IBD).

h. **Rheumatoid Arthritis**

Rheumatoid joint inflammation (RA) is a constant fiery problem that essentially influences the joints. In RA, the resistant framework goes after the synovium, the covering of the films that encompass the joints. This prompts Inflammation, thickening of the synovium, and harm to the ligament and bones inside the joints.

The ongoing Inflammation in RA results from the determined presence of safe cells and favorable to fiery cytokines in the joints. These fiery middle people advance the enrollment of extra safe cells and sustain the pattern of Inflammation and joint obliteration. Overseeing Inflammation is a vital part of RA treatment, frequently including meds like nonsteroidal calming drugs (NSAIDs), corticosteroids, and illness-changing antirheumatic drugs (DMARDs).

i. **Lupus**

Fundamental lupus erythematosus (SLE), usually known as lupus, is an immune system sickness that can influence various organs and frameworks in the body. Lupus is portrayed by the development of auto-antibodies, which focus on the body's cells and tissues. This prompts inescapable Inflammation and harm to organs like the kidneys, heart, lungs, and skin.

The specific reason for lupus isn't completely perceived, yet it is accepted to include a blend of hereditary, natural, and hormonal elements. Ongoing aggravation in lupus is driven by the tenacious actuation of the safe framework and the creation of fiery cytokines. Overseeing lupus includes decreasing Inflammation and smothering the invulnerable reaction to forestall organ harm.

j.   **Fiery Entrail Illness (IBD)**

Incendiary gut infection (IBD) incorporates conditions, for example, Crohn's illness and ulcerative colitis, which are portrayed by persistent aggravation of the gastrointestinal (GI) parcel. In IBD, the resistant framework erroneously focuses on the cells covering the digestive organs, prompting Inflammation, ulcers, and harm to the GI lot.

The ongoing Inflammation in IBD upsets the typical working of the gut-related framework, causing side effects like gut torment, runs, weight reduction, and weariness. Overseeing Inflammation is a focal part of IBD treatment and may include meds like corticosteroids, immunosuppressant, and biologics, as well as dietary and way-of-life Transformations.

k.   **Malignant growth**

Persistent Inflammation is progressively perceived as a contributing component in the turn of events and movement of specific kinds of disease. Provocative cells and go-betweens can advance cancer development, intrusion, and metastasis.

Inflammation and Disease Development

Inflammation can add to disease advancement through a few instruments:

1. **DNA Damage:** Provocative cells produce responsive oxygen species (ROS) and receptive nitrogen species(RNS) as a feature of the insusceptible reaction. These receptive atoms can cause DNA harm and transformations, which can prompt the improvement of disease.

2. **Proliferation and Survival:** Fiery arbiters, for example, cytokines and development elements can advance the multiplication and endurance of malignant growth cells. They make a microenvironment that upholds growth development and shields disease cells from resistant observation.

3. **Angiogenesis**: Persistent aggravation can invigorate angiogenesis, the development of fresh blood vessels. Cancers require a blood supply to develop and spread, and angiogenesis gives the essential supplements and oxygen for growth movement.

4. **Metastasis**: Fiery middle people can upgrade the capacity of disease cells to attack encompassing tissues and spread to far-off destinations (metastasis). This cycle is worked with by chemicals that corrupt the extracellular framework and by flagging pathways that advance cell relocation.

Instances of Inflammation-Related Cancers

Particular sorts of disease are firmly connected with persistent aggravation:

- ✓ **Colorectal Cancer:** Persistent Inflammation in the colon, as found in conditions like ulcerative colitis and

Crohn's illness, builds the gamble of colorectal disease. The continuous Inflammation prompts DNA harm, cell multiplication, and Transformations in the gut microbiota, all of which add to malignant growth advancement.

✓ **Liver Cancer:** Ongoing aggravation of the liver, frequently coming about because of persistent hepatitis B or C diseases or conditions like non-alcoholic steatohepatitis (NASH), expands the gamble of liver malignant growth (hepatocellular carcinoma). The relentless provocative reaction harms liver cells and advances the improvement of malignant cells.

✓ **Gut Cancer:** Constant contamination with Helicobacter pylori microscopic organisms can prompt long haul aggravation of the gut lining (gastritis), expanding the gamble of gut disease. The aggravation brought about by H. pylori can bring about Transformations to the gut cells, advancing disease improvement.

✓ **Neurodegenerative Infections:** Constant aggravation is likewise embroiled in the turn of events and movement of neurodegenerative sicknesses, like Alzheimer's illness and Parkinson's infection. Inflammation in the mind can prompt the amassing of harmful proteins, neuronal harm, and weakened mental capability.

✓ **Alzheimer's Disease:** Alzheimer's sickness is described by the collection of amyloid-beta plaques and tau tangles in the cerebrum. These unusual protein stores trigger an

CHAPTER 2: The Gut-Inflammation Connection

2.11 The Gut Microbiome

The human gut/gut is home to trillions of microorganisms, including microscopic organisms, infections, growths, and different organisms. This different local area of organic entities, on the whole, known as the gut microbiome, assumes a pivotal part in keeping up with generally speaking well-being and prosperity. Late exploration has featured the huge effect of the gut microbiome on aggravation and its capability to impact different medical issues. Understanding the gut microbiome and its association with aggravation can give experiences into the anticipation and the board of persistent illnesses.

What is the gut Microbiome?

The gut microbiome is a mind-boggling environment of microorganisms that live in the gastrointestinal (GI) lot. These microorganisms are principally tracked down in the digestive organs, especially in the colon. The organization of the gut microbiome is remarkable to every person and is affected by different variables, including hereditary qualities, diet, climate, and way of life.

The gut microbiome comprises a few kinds of microorganisms:

- ❖ **Bacteria:** The most bountiful and all-around concentrated on individuals from the gut microbiome. Normal bacterial phyla incorporate Firmicutes, Bacteroidetes, Actinobacteria, and Proteobacteria.
- ❖ **Viruses:** Infections that contaminate microbes (bacteriophages) and eukaryotic cells are available in the gut.

- ❖ **Fungi:** Yeasts and molds are additionally essential for the gut microbiome, even though they are available in more modest numbers contrasted with microscopic organisms.
- ❖ **Archaea:** An unmistakable gathering of microorganisms that are like microscopic organisms yet have exceptional qualities.

The gut microbiome carries out a few fundamental roles that are basic for keeping up with well-being:

1. Digesting Food: Gut microorganisms assist with separating complex carbs, strands, and other unpalatable parts of the eating regimen, creating short-chain unsaturated fats (SCFAs) and different metabolites that give energy and supplements to the host.

2. Synthesizing Vitamins: Certain gut microorganisms combine fundamental nutrients, for example, vitamin K and B nutrients, which are significant for different physiological capabilities.

3. **Regulating Resistant Function:** The gut microbiome assumes an essential part in the turn of events and guidelines of the safe framework. It helps train the invulnerable framework to recognize innocuous and hurtful substances.

4. **Protecting against Pathogens:** The gut microbiome acts as a hindrance against pathogenic microorganisms by viewing for assets and delivering antimicrobial substances.

5. **Modulating Inflammation**: Gut microorganisms can impact fiery cycles by communicating with the insusceptible framework and delivering metabolites that have mitigating or favorable to incendiary impacts.

The Gut-Inflammation Connection

The connection between the gut microbiome and aggravation is perplexing and bidirectional. The gut microbiome can impact aggravation, and Inflammation can, thus, influence the piece and capability of the gut microbiome. This perplexing transaction has critical ramifications for well-being and illness.

Gut Dysbiosis and Inflammation

Gut dysbiosis alludes to a lopsidedness or disturbance in the creation of the gut microbiome. Dysbiosis can result from different elements, including terrible eating routines, anti-infection use, stress, and diseases. At the point when the equilibrium of the gut microbiome is upset, it can prompt expanded aggravation and add to the advancement of constant sicknesses.

Instruments Connecting Gut Dysbiosis to Inflammation

A few instruments make sense of how gut dysbiosis can advance Inflammation:

1. Increased Digestive Permeability: Gut dysbiosis can prompt expanded gastrointestinal penetrability, frequently alluded to as "defective gut." The gastrointestinal coating is a significant hindrance that keeps destructive substances from entering the circulation system. At the point when this hindrance is compromised, poisons, microorganisms, and undigested food particles can spill into the circulatory system, setting off an insusceptible reaction and fundamental Inflammation.

2. Altered Safe Responses: The gut microbiome associates with the invulnerable framework through different flagging pathways. Dysbiosis can upset these associations, prompting an unevenness in safe reactions. For instance, certain gut microorganisms produce metabolites like SCFAs that make calming impacts. A decrease in these useful microscopic organisms can bring about expanded Inflammation.

3. Production of Supportive Fiery Metabolites: Some gut microorganisms produce metabolites that advance aggravation. For instance, lipopolysaccharides (LPS), parts of the external film of specific microscopic organisms, can set off areas of strength for a reaction and Inflammation when they enter the circulatory system.

4. Imbalanced Microbial Metabolites: Dysbiosis can modify the creation of microbial metabolites that manage Inflammation. Awkwardness in these metabolites can advance ongoing aggravation. For example, a reduction in SCFAs, which have calming properties, can prompt expanded Inflammation.

Conditions Related to Gut Dysbiosis and Inflammation

A few persistent medical issues have been connected to destroying dysbiosis and Inflammation:

1. Inflammatory Entrail Illness (IBD): IBD, including Crohn's sickness and ulcerative colitis, is portrayed by the persistent aggravation of the GI parcel. Research has shown that people with IBD have particular adjustments in their gut microbiome, including decreased variety and an irregularity among helpful and hurtful microscopic organisms.

2. Metabolic Disorders: Corpulence and type 2 diabetes are related to gut dysbiosis and constant poor-quality aggravation. Investigations have discovered that people with these circumstances frequently have a modified gut microbiome organization, which might add to insulin opposition and metabolic brokenness.

3. Cardiovascular Disease: Ongoing Inflammation is vital to consider the improvement of atherosclerosis and cardiovascular illness. Gut dysbiosis can add to fundamental aggravation, which thusly advances the development of atherosclerotic plaques.

4. Autoimmune Diseases: Immune system illnesses, like rheumatoid joint inflammation, various sclerosis, and lupus, include a safe reaction against the body's tissues. Gut dysbiosis has been embroiled in the pathogenesis of these illnesses, possibly by influencing safe guidelines and advancing Inflammation.

5. Neurological Disorders: Arising research recommends that the gut microbiome may assume a part in neurological circumstances like Alzheimer's sickness, Parkinson's illness, and mental imbalance range problems. Inflammation and insusceptible reactions impacted by the gut microbiome may add to the turn of events and movement of these circumstances.

Regulating the Gut Microbiome to Lessen Aggravation

Given the critical effect of the gut microbiome on Inflammation and well-being, systems to balance the gut microbiome are being investigated as expected restorative methodologies. Here are far to advance a solid gut microbiome and diminish Inflammation:

Dietary Interventions

1. Fiber-Rich Diet: An eating regimen high in fiber advances the development of helpful gut microorganisms that produce SCFAs, which have mitigating properties. Food sources wealthy in fiber incorporate organic products, vegetables, entire grains, vegetables, and nuts.

2. Probiotics: Probiotics are live microorganisms that give medical advantages when consumed in satisfactory sums. They can assist with re-establishing a good arrangement of gut microorganisms and lessen the Inflammation. Probiotic-rich food sources incorporate yogurt, kefir, sauerkraut, kimchi, and other matured food varieties. Probiotic supplements are likewise accessible.

3. Prebiotics: Prebiotics are non-edible strands that act as nourishment for advantageous gut microscopic organisms. They advance the development and action of these microorganisms. Prebiotic-rich food sources incorporate garlic, onions, leeks, asparagus, bananas, and chicory root.

4. Anti-Incendiary Foods: Integrating mitigating food varieties into the eating regimen can assist with lessening Inflammation. These food varieties incorporate greasy fish (rich in omega-3 unsaturated fats), berries, salad greens, nuts, seeds, olive oil, and turmeric.

Way of life Modifications

1. Regular Actual Activity: Exercise has been displayed to advance a sound gut microbiome and lessen Inflammation. Customary actual work can build the variety of gut microscopic organisms and improve the creation of mitigating metabolites.

2. Stress Management: Persistent pressure can adversely affect the gut microbiome and advance Inflammation. Stress-decreasing strategies like care reflection, yoga, profound breathing activities, and sufficient rest can assist with keeping a solid gut microbiome.

3. Avoiding Superfluous Antibiotics: While anti-toxins are fundamental for treating bacterial contaminations, their abuse can disturb the gut microbiome. It is essential to utilize anti-

infection agents reasonably and just when endorsed by a medical services professional.

Arising Therapies

1. Fecal Microbiota Transplantation (FMT): FMT includes moving stool from a sound benefactor to the GI plot of a beneficiary with gut dysbiosis. This strategy plans to reestablish a solid gut microbiome and has shown guarantee in treating conditions, for example, repetitive Clostridioides difficile contamination and fiery gut sickness.

2. Microbiome-Designated Drugs: Specialists are creating drugs that explicitly focus on the gut microbiome to tweak aggravation and treat constant sicknesses. These medications might incorporate prebiotics, probiotics, postbiotics (metabolites delivered by gut microorganisms), and other microbiome-adjusting specialists.

3. Personalized Nutrition: Advances in microbiome research are preparing for customized nourishment plans in light of a singular's one-of-kind gut microbiome profile. Customized sustenance means to upgrade gut well-being and lessening aggravation by fitting dietary proposals to the person's microbiome

2.12 How Gut Health Affects Inflammation

The gut, frequently alluded to as the "second cerebrum," is a perplexing biological system containing trillions of microorganisms that assume an urgent part in keeping up with generally speaking well-being. Past its part in assimilation, the gut impacts different physiological cycles, including safe capability and Inflammation. The late examination has revealed insight into the mind-boggling connection between gut wellbeing and Inflammation, uncovering how disturbances in the gut microbiome can add to persistent aggravation and the advancement of various medical issues.

Figuring out the Gut Microbiome

The gut microbiome alludes to the assorted local area of microorganisms that occupy the gastrointestinal lot, dominatingly the internal organ. This microbial environment incorporates microscopic organisms, infections, growths, and archaea, which aggregately communicate with the host's cells and assume fundamental parts in assimilation, digestion, and resistance capability.

Arrangement of the Gut Microbiome

The arrangement of the gut microbiome is affected by different elements, including hereditary qualities, diet, age, geology, and drug use. While there is critical relational variety, certain bacterial phyla, like Firmicutes and Bacteroidetes, rule the gut microbiome in solid people. These microbes carry out basic roles, like maturing dietary fiber to create short-chain unsaturated fats (SCFAs) like butyrate, acetic acid derivation, and propionate, which give energy to digestive cells and apply mitigating impacts.

Job of Gut Microbiome in Safe Regulation

The gut microbiome plays a critical part in controlling resistant reactions. Gut microscopic organisms connect intimately with resistant cells in the gut-related lymphoid tissue (GALT), affecting the turn of events and capability of the safe framework. This collaboration is essential for keeping up with resistant resilience — where the invulnerable framework perceives and endures innocuous antigens while mounting vigorous reactions against microorganisms.

Gut Wellbeing and Inflammation

Inflammation is an essential resistant reaction intended to shield the body from contamination and injury. Notwithstanding, when Inflammation becomes persistent and dysregulated, it can add to the pathogenesis of different sicknesses. The gut microbiome applies a significant effect on Inflammation through a few systems, featuring its essential job in keeping up with resistant homeostasis.

1. Gastrointestinal Obstruction Integrity

The gastrointestinal epithelium fills in as an actual obstruction that specifically permits supplements and water to pass while forestalling the section of unsafe substances, including microorganisms and poisons, into the foundational course. Disturbances in digestive boundary trustworthiness, generally alluded to as "defective gut," can happen due to dysbiosis — the lopsidedness of gut microbial networks. Dysbiosis can prompt expanded digestive penetrability, permitting bacterial parts, for example, lipopolysaccharides (LPS), to move into the circulatory system and trigger foundational Inflammation.

2. Creation of Short-Chain Unsaturated fats (SCFAs)

Short-chain unsaturated fats (SCFAs), dominatingly created through the maturation of dietary fiber by gut microorganisms, assume a basic part in balancing Inflammation. Butyrate, specifically, has strong calming properties by hindering the atomic element kappa B (NF-κB) pathway — a vital controller of fiery reactions in safe cells. SCFAs likewise advance the age of administrative Lymphocytes (Tregs), which stifle exorbitant resistant enactment and keep up with insusceptible resilience.

3. Guideline of Invulnerable Responses

Gut microbes cooperate with safe cells through different flagging pathways, impacting the harmony between supportive incendiary and mitigating reactions. Commensal microbes animate the creation of calming cytokines, like interleukin-10 (IL-10), while restraining the discharge of supportive of incendiary cytokines, including growth putrefaction factor-alpha (TNF-α) and interleukin-6 (IL-6). Lopsided characteristics in the gut microbiome organization can upset this sensitive safe guideline, prompting ongoing Inflammation and immune system illnesses.

4. Metabolite Production

In past SCFAs, gut microscopic organisms produce a horde of metabolites that affect physiology and Inflammation. These metabolites incorporate synapses, bile acids, and optional bile acids, which can adjust resistant cell capability and provocative pathways. For example, optional bile acids restrain the actuation of NF-κB and mitogen-enacted protein kinase (MAPK) flagging pathways, accordingly diminishing aggravation in the gut and foundationally.

Gut Dysbiosis and Fiery Infections

Dysbiosis, described by Transformations in gut microbiome structure and capability, has been ensnared in the pathogenesis of various fiery illnesses. Understanding the job of gut dysbiosis in advancing aggravation gives experiences into potential remedial systems pointed toward reestablishing microbial equilibrium and reducing illness side effects.

1. Fiery Inside Infection (IBD)

Fiery inside infection (IBD), including Crohn's illness and ulcerative colitis, is described by constant Inflammation of the gastrointestinal plot. Studies have distinguished dysbiosis in people with IBD, described by decreased microbial variety, consumption of gainful microscopic organisms, and extension of possibly pathogenic species. This dysbiosis adds to digestive boundary brokenness, distorted invulnerable actuation, and supported aggravation, propagating sickness movement.

2. Metabolic Condition and Obesity

Corpulence and metabolic conditions are related to poor quality ongoing Inflammation, adding to insulin obstruction, dyslipidemia, and cardiovascular sickness. Dysbiosis in corpulent people is portrayed by an expanded proportion of Firmicutes to Bacteroidetes, adjusted SCFA creation, and improved gut porousness. These progressions advance fundamental aggravation, fat tissue brokenness, and metabolic aggravations, featuring the job of gut microbiome dysregulation in metabolic illnesses.

3. Immune System Disorders

Immune system problems, for example, rheumatoid joint inflammation, fundamental lupus erythematosus (SLE), and various sclerosis (MS), result from resistant-intervened assaults on self-tissues. Dysbiosis can set off immune system reactions by disturbing resistant resilience components and advancing fiery cytokine creation. For instance, certain gut microbes produce antigens that copy proteins, prompting cross-receptive resistant reactions and tissue harm in defenseless people.

4. Neurological and Mental Disorders

Arising proof recommends a connection between gut dysbiosis and neurological issues, including Alzheimer's sickness, Parkinson's illness, and misery. Dysbiosis-actuated Inflammation might add to neuro-inflammation, neuronal brokenness, and mental weakness through microbial metabolites, invulnerable dysregulation, and vagus nerve flagging. Tweaking the gut microbiome addresses a likely restorative methodology for overseeing neurological and mental circumstances by relieving Inflammation and reestablishing microbial equilibrium.

Restorative Ways to Deal and Regulate Gut Wellbeing and Inflammation

Given the basic job of the gut microbiome in managing Inflammation, remedial systems pointed toward reestablishing microbial equilibrium and advancing gut well-being stand out. These methodologies incorporate dietary intercessions, probiotics, prebiotics, transplantation (FMT), and designated pharmacological specialists intended to regulate microbial organization and capability.

1. Dietary Interventions

An eating routine wealthy in fiber, entire grains, organic products, and vegetables advances microbial variety and SCFA creation, in this manner moderating Inflammation and upgrading gut hindrance uprightness. On the other hand, high-fat weight control plans and unreasonable sugar admission have been related to dysbiosis, gut porousness, and foundational aggravation, highlighting the significance of dietary quality in keeping up with gut well-being.

2. Probiotics and Prebiotics

Probiotics, live microorganisms that present medical advantages when managed in sufficient sums, apply calming impacts by tweaking safe reactions and advancing microbial variety. Prebiotics, non-edible filaments that act as substrates for useful microscopic organisms, animate SCFA creation and upgrade gut obstruction capability, consequently decreasing Inflammation and supporting resistant homeostasis.

3. Waste Microbiota Transplantation (FMT)

FMT includes moving waste material from a solid benefactor to a beneficiary with dysbiosis-related messes, for example, intermittent Clostridioides difficile disease and ulcerative colitis. FMT reestablishes microbial variety, improves SCFA creation, and stifles pathogenic microscopic organisms, along these lines easing aggravation and advancing illness reduction in select patient populations.

4. Microbiome-Designated Therapeutics

Propels in microbiome research have worked with the improvement of microbiome-designated drugs intended to tweak microbial synthesis and capability. These incorporate postbiotics, microbial-inferred metabolites that apply calming impacts, and designed probiotics fit for conveying restorative specialists to target destinations inside the gastrointestinal parcel. Such mediations hold a guarantee for the accuracy of medication approaches custom-fitted to individual microbiome profiles and infection states.

Future Headings in Gut Microbiome Exploration

The prospering field of gut microbiome research keeps on disentangling the unpredictable transaction between microbial networks, physiology, and sickness pathogenesis. Future examinations expect to clarify microbiome-have cooperations, distinguish microbial biomarkers of sickness chance and movement, and foster customized mediations to reestablish gut well-being and lighten Inflammation.

1. Accuracy Nourishment and Customized Medicine

Progresses in metagenomics and multi-omics advances empower thorough profiling of gut microbiome synthesis, practical potential, and metabolic exercises. Incorporating microbiome information with clinical boundaries works with the advancement of customized nourishment designs and designated treatments custom-made to individual microbial profiles and well-being results.

2. Restorative Applications in Constant Diseases

The restorative capability of gut microbiome-designated mediations reaches out past gastrointestinal issues including metabolic illnesses, immune system problems, neurodegenerative infections, and mental problems. Tackling microbial biomarkers and restorative specialists offers novel techniques to moderate aggravation, reestablish safe homeostasis, and work on understanding results across different infection settings.

3. Cross-Disciplinary Coordinated Efforts and Translational Research

Coordinated efforts between microbiologists, immunologists, clinicians, and computational scholars are fundamental for progressing translational examination and clinical applications in gut microbiome science. Coordinating essential science disclosures with clinical preliminaries and patient-focused results works with the interpretation of microbiome-based treatments into clinical work, making ready for accurate medication approaches in medical care.

2.13 Indications of an Unhealthy Gut

A solid gut is vital for general prosperity, impacting processing, safe capability, and, surprisingly, emotional well-being. On the other hand, an unfortunate gut, described by dysbiosis and Inflammation, can prompt a scope of side effects and add to the improvement of constant infections. Perceiving the indications of an unfortunate gut is urgent for early intercession and advancing gut well-being. This part investigates normal signs and side effects of gut brokenness, featuring the many-sided connection between gut well-being and aggravation.

1. **Prologue to Destroy Wellbeing**

The gut, frequently referred to as the gastrointestinal lot, incorporates the gut, small digestive tract, and internal organs (colon). It fills in as a vital connection point between the outer climate and the interior milieu, liable for processing, supplement retention, and resistant observation. Fundamental to destroying well-being is the gut microbiome — a different local area of microorganisms that live inside the digestive lumen.

2. **Grasping the Gut Microbiome**

The gut microbiome contains trillions of microorganisms, including microscopic organisms, infections, growths, and archaea, which aggregately add to digestion, resistant guidelines, and insurance against microorganisms. The arrangement of the gut microbiome is affected by variables like eating regimen, drugs, way of life, and natural openings. In a solid expression, the gut microbiome keeps a sensitive equilibrium, advancing beneficial interaction between commensal (helpful) and possibly pathogenic microscopic organisms.

Indications of an Undesirable Gut

1. Digestive Issues

Gut-related side effects are among the most widely recognized signs of gut brokenness. These side effects might include:

a. Ongoing Blockage or Diarrhea: Determined Transformations in entrail propensities, like rare defecations or diarrheas, may imply adjustments in gut motility and microbial structure.

b. Gas **and Bloating:** Inordinate gas creation and swelling following feasts can show weakened absorption and aging of undigested starches by gut microorganisms.

c. **Reflux and Heartburn:** Gastro-esophageal reflux sickness (GERD) and indigestion might result from dysregulation of esophageal sphincter capability or adjustments in gastric corrosive creation.

d. Gut **Torment or Cramping:** Repetitive gut inconvenience, squeezing, or fits might go with fiery circumstances, like touchy entrail disorder (IBS) or incendiary inside sickness (IBD).

2. Food Bigotries and Sensitivities

People with an undesirable gut might encounter increased aversion to specific food varieties, prompting side effects, for example,

- ❖ **Food Intolerances:** Failure to process explicit food sources, like lactose narrow-mindedness (because of lack of lactase protein) or gluten prejudice (celiac illness).
- ❖ **Food Sensitivities:** Non-hypersensitive resistant reactions to food parts, setting off side effects like migraines, skin rashes, or gastrointestinal distress.

3. Unintentional Weight Transformations

Transformations in body weight, especially accidental weight reduction or gain, may reflect basic metabolic aggravations related to gut dysbiosis and Inflammation.

4. Fatigue and Low Energy

Ongoing weariness and lessened energy levels can result from weakened supplement retention, adjusted digestion, or fundamental Inflammation related with gut brokenness.

5. Mental Wellbeing Symptoms

The gut mind pivot — a complex correspondence network between the gut microbiome and the focal sensory system — assumes an essential part in directing temperament and mental capability. Indications of an undesirable gut influencing emotional well-being might include:

- **Mindset Disorders:** Expanded nervousness, gloom, or emotional episodes might connect with dysbiosis-actuated aggravation and Transformations in synapse creation.
- Mental Impairment: Unfortunate focus, memory slips, or mind haze could come from neuro-inflammatory reactions interceded by gut-inferred metabolites.

6. Skin Conditions

Skin well-being is unpredictably connected to destroying respectability and microbial equilibrium. Normal skin indications of gut brokenness include:

- **Acne**: Constant Inflammation and dysbiosis can worsen skin break-out vulgaris through foundational invulnerable enactment and adjusted sebum creation.

- **Dermatitis and Psoriasis**: Incendiary skin problems might be affected by invulnerable dysregulation set off by gut-determined antigens and cytokines.

7. Autoimmune Disorders

Immune system infections emerge from dysregulated invulnerable reactions focusing on self-tissues. Gut brokenness and expanded digestive penetrability (defective gut) may add to immune system conditions, for example,

- **Rheumatoid Arthritis**: Joint aggravation and ligament annihilation connected to autoantibody creation set off by gut dysbiosis.
- **Hashimoto's Thyroiditis:** Immune system thyroid illness described by lymphocytic invasion of the thyroid organ, possibly impacted by gut intervened insusceptible actuation.

8. Chronic Fiery Conditions

Foundational Inflammation originating from an unfortunate gut can incline people toward constant provocative illnesses, including:

- **Cardiovascular Disease:** Atherosclerosis and coronary course illness exacerbated by constant second-rate aggravation and dyslipidemia.
- **Metabolic Syndrome:** Insulin obstruction, dyslipidemia, and focal heftiness related to fundamental Inflammation and Transformation adipokine creation.

Instruments of Gut-Related Inflammation

The signs and side effects of an undesirable gut are unpredictably connected to dysbiosis-incited Inflammation and insusceptible dysregulation. Key instruments to destroy related Inflammation include:

1. Intestinal Boundary Dysfunction

- Flawed Gut Syndrome: Expanded digestive penetrability permits bacterial endotoxins (e.g., lipopolysaccharides, LPS) and undigested food particles to move into the foundational course, setting off safe reactions and fundamental aggravation.

2. Altered Invulnerable Responses

- Invulnerable Activation: Dysbiosis disturbs resistant homeostasis, advancing supportive of incendiary cytokine creation (e.g., TNF-α, IL-6) and impeding mitigating systems (e.g., Treg cell capability).

3. Microbial Metabolites

- Short-Chain Unsaturated fats (SCFAs): Decreased SCFA creation from fiber aging lessens calming flagging and mucosal hindrance uprightness, fueling Gut-related Inflammation.

4. Neuroimmune Interactions

- Gut Mind Axis: Bidirectional correspondence between the gut microbiome and the focal sensory system impacts synapse blend (e.g., serotonin) and temperament guideline, influencing emotional wellness results.

Indicative Methodologies and Treatment Techniques

Distinguishing indications of an unfortunate gut include far-reaching assessment of side effects, dietary propensities, clinical history, and demonstrative testing. Symptomatic methodologies might include:

- Stool Analysis: Surveying microbial variety, microorganism presence, and fiery markers (e.g., calprotectin) to portray gut dysbiosis and aggravation.

- Food End Diet: Distinguishing food triggers and bigotries through precise end and renewed introduction of suspect food sources.

- Blood Tests: Estimating provocative markers (e.g., C-receptive protein, cytokines) and immune system antibodies to assess fundamental aggravation and insusceptible initiation.

Advancing Gut Wellbeing and Decreasing Inflammation

Viable administration of gut-related Inflammation centers on reestablishing microbial equilibrium, upgrading gut boundary uprightness, and regulating safe reactions through designated mediations:

1. Probiotics and Prebiotics: Enhancing with useful microorganisms (probiotics) and non-edible filaments (prebiotics) advances microbial variety, SCFA creation, and invulnerable resistance.

2. Dietary Modifications: Embracing a different, fiber-rich eating regimen rich in organic products, vegetables, entire grains, and

matured food varieties upholds gut well-being and mitigates Inflammation.

3. Stress Management: Rehearsing pressure decrease procedures (e.g., care, yoga) and enhancing rest examples to limit neuroendocrine pressure reactions and backing gut mind pivot balance.

4. Medication Management: Working intimately with medical care suppliers to prudently utilize anti-microbial, non-steroidal mitigating drugs (NSAIDs), and different prescriptions influencing gut microbiota and Inflammation.

CHAPTER 3: Getting Ready for Your Transformation

3.11 Putting forth Practical Objectives

Leaving on an excursion of Transformation ,whether it's further developing well-being, accomplishing wellness achievements, or upgrading generally speaking prosperity starts with laying out reasonable and reachable objectives. Laying out objectives gives guidance, inspiration, and a structure for estimating progress en route. In this section, we dive into the significance of objective setting in your Transformation process, methodologies for laying out practical objectives, and how to remain focused on accomplishing them.

Figuring out the Force of Objectives

Objectives act as directing reference points that impel people toward wanted results, cultivating clearness, concentration, and responsibility all through the Transformation cycle. Whether you want to get fitter from muscle, embrace better dietary patterns, or lessen feelings of anxiety, defining clear and sensible objectives establishes the groundwork for progress.

Advantages of Objective Setting

1. **Clarity and Focus:** characterized objectives explain your vision and give a guide to activity, assisting you with focusing on errands and dispensing se assets successfully.

2. **Motivation and Commitment:** Objectives light natural inspiration and responsibility, filling perseverance and versatility notwithstanding difficulties and misfortunes.

3. **Measurable Progress:** Laying out quantifiable objectives permits you to follow progress equitably, celebrate

accomplishments, and Transformation procedures on a case-by-case basis to remain on track.

4. **Accountability and Responsibility**: Objectives create a feeling of responsibility, empowering moral obligation regarding activities and results connected with your Transformation process.

Standards of Compelling Objective Setting

Compelling objective setting includes adjusting goals to reasonable assumptions and significant stages. By applying these standards, you can make objectives that are significant, achievable, and helpful for practical Transformation:

1. **Specificity**: Characterize your objectives with lucidity and explicitness, framing what you need to accomplish, why it makes a difference, and the means expected to arrive at your ideal result. For instance, rather than laying out a dubious objective like "get thinner," determine an objective weight reduction sum (e.g., 10 pounds) and period (e.g., 90 days).

2. **Measurability:** Lay out rules for estimating progress and achievement. Whether following body estimations, wellness achievements, dietary Transformations, or feelings of anxiety, quantifiable measurements give unmistakable signs of progress and regions for development.

3. **Achievability:** Put forth objectives that are testing yet achievable inside your ongoing capacities and assets. Think about your assets, impediments, and accessible emotionally supportive networks while characterizing the degree and timetable of your objectives.

5. **Time-bound**: Lay out a sensible period for accomplishing every objective, consolidating cutoff times and achievements to

keep up with concentration and energy. Separating bigger objectives into more modest, reasonable assignments improves responsibility and works with consistent advancement after some time.

Kinds of Transformation Objectives

Transformation objectives incorporate different aspects of self-awareness and prosperity, enveloping physical, mental, profound, and otherworldly aspects. Consider these classifications while putting forth objectives customized to your interesting Transformation venture:

1. Physical Wellbeing and Fitness

- ✓ Weight Management: Defining objectives for weight reduction, muscle gain, or body piece enhancements given sensible courses of events and feasible methodologies (e.g., adjusted sustenance, standard activity).
- ✓ **Actual Performance:** Laying out objectives for working on cardiovascular perseverance, strength, adaptability, or athletic execution through organized preparing projects and moderate over-burden standards.
- ✓ Nourishing Habits: Embracing objectives to develop better dietary patterns, like expanding products of the soil admission, decreasing handled food varieties, and careful eating rehearses.

2. Mental and close to home Well-being

- ❖ Stress Management: Defining objectives to lessen feelings of anxiety through unwinding procedures, care rehearses, and powerful time usage systems.
- ❖ Mental Enhancement: Laying out objectives for improving mental capability, memory, and mental

clearness through cerebrum preparing works, instructive pursuits, or invigorating exercises.

❖ Profound Resilience: Creating objectives to develop close-to-home versatility and versatile survival techniques because of life difficulties, misfortunes, and advances.

3. Lifestyle and Social Transformations

➢ Rest Optimization: Laying out objectives to further develop rest quality and length through rest cleanliness rehearses, sleep time schedules, and stress decrease methods.

➢ Actual work Integration: Laying out objectives to integrate customary active work into day-to-day schedules, for example, strolling breaks, work area activities, or dynamic driving.

Substance Use Reduction: Taking on objectives to lessen or dispose of unsafe substance use ways of behaving, like smoking suspension, liquor balance, or caffeine admission to the board.

4. Relationships and Social Connections

• Social Engagement: Putting forth objectives to support significant connections, grow interpersonal organizations, and partake in local area exercises or volunteer drives.

• Correspondence Skills: Creating objectives to improve correspondence adequacy, undivided attention abilities, and compromise methodologies in private and expert connections.

• Limits and Self-Care: Laying out objectives to lay out solid limits, focus on taking care of oneself practices, and develop strong conditions helpful for self-awareness and prosperity.

Techniques for Objective Accomplishment

Accomplishing Transformation objectives requires proactive preparation, diligence, and a promise to persistent improvement. Carry out these procedures to upgrade objective accomplishment and streamline your Transformation process:

1. **Create an Activity Plan:** Separate bigger objectives into more modest, sensible activity ventures with clear cutoff times and achievements. Foster an organized activity plan illustrating explicit undertakings, assets required, and responsibility measures.

2. **Monitor Progress:** Consistently survey progress toward your objectives utilizing objective measurements, journaling, or following applications. Celebrate accomplishments; distinguish regions for development, and Transformation methodologies on a case-by-case basis to remain on track.

3. **Seek Backing and Accountability:** Draw in tutors, mentors, or steady friends who can give direction, support, and productive criticism all through your Transformation process. Joining support gatherings or online networks can likewise encourage kinship and shared encounters.

5. **Celebrate Milestones:** Recognize and celebrate achievements, regardless of how little, to support progress, help inspire, and support force toward accomplishing bigger objectives. Think about accomplishments, examples learned, and self-awareness encounters en route.

Defeating Normal Difficulties

Exploring the way toward transformation

Exploring the way toward Transformation unavoidably presents difficulties and hindrances that might test your determination and flexibility. By expecting normal difficulties and carrying out proactive methodologies, you can conquer hindrances and keep up with force toward accomplishing your objectives:

1. Time Constraints: Focus on using time productively and designate devoted time allotments for objective-related exercises. Break undertakings into more modest augmentations, delegate liabilities whenever the situation allows, and smooth out schedules to enhance efficiency.

2. Self-Uncertainty and Negative Self-Talk: Develop self-sympathy, positive confirmations, and a development mentality to balance self-restricting convictions and negative idea designs. Encircle yourself with steady people who elevate and energize your advancement.

3. Plateaus and Setbacks: Embrace mishaps as learning opens doors and amazing open doors for development. Reconsider objectives, Transformation systems, and look for direction from guides or specialists to conquer levels and recapture energy toward accomplishing wanted results.

4. Lack of Motivation: Reconnect with your inborn inspirations, return to your objectives and desires, and imagine the advantages of accomplishing Transformation achievements. Integrate persuasive methods, for example, perception works out, objective setting customs, or rousing updates, to reignite energy and responsibility.

3.12 Fundamental Devices and Fixings

Leaving on a Transformation venture requires something other than inspiration; it requires the right instruments and fixings to uphold your objectives. Whether you're expecting to upgrade your actual wellness, embrace better dietary patterns, or develop a more adjusted way of life, outfitting yourself with fundamental instruments and fixings makes way for progress. This part investigates the key parts expected to advance your Transformation process, enabling you to accomplish feasible and significant Transformation.

The Groundwork of Transformation

The Transformation includes complex parts of self-awareness, incorporating physical, mental, profound, and otherworldly aspects. To successfully explore this excursion, consider the accompanying fundamental components for getting ready and supporting your Transformation endeavors

1. Mindset and Motivation

Accomplishing enduring Transformation starts with developing a positive outlook and natural inspiration lined up with your objectives. Your mentality shapes your convictions, perspectives, and ways of behaving, affecting your capacity to conquer difficulties and remain focused on your Transformation process.

> **Care Practices:** Consolidate care methods, like contemplation, profound breathing activities, or representation, to improve mindfulness, center, and close-to-home flexibility.
> **Objective Visualization:** Imagine your ideal results and imagine the advantages of accomplishing Transformation achievements. Perception strategies can

build up inspiration, explain expectations, and fortify obligation to your objectives.

➢ **Insistences and Positive Self-Talk:** Take on confirmations and positive self-converse with challenge self-restricting convictions, help fearlessness, and develop a development situated outlook helpful for self-awareness.

2. Goal-Setting and Planning

Setting clear, sensible, and noteworthy objectives gives a guide to your Transformation process, directing your endeavors and estimating progress en route. Successful objective-setting techniques include:

✓ **Shrewd Goals:** Characterize objectives that are Explicit, Quantifiable, Attainable, Applicable, and Time-bound. Brilliant standards upgrade objective clearness, responsibility, and possibility, working with consistent advancement and inspiration.

✓ **Activity Plans:** Foster organized activity plans to frame bit-bit assignments, timetables, and assets expected to accomplish every objective. Separating bigger objectives into reasonable activity steps advances consistency, concentration, and energy.

✓ **Following and Monitoring:** Execute the following components, for example, journaling, progress outlines, or computerized applications, to screen objective advancement, celebrate accomplishments, and recognize regions for Transformation or improvement.

3. Nutrition and Dietary Habits

Streamlining sustenance frames a foundation of actual well-being and imperativeness, giving fundamental supplements to help cell capability, energy digestion, and in general prosperity. Key contemplations for upgrading dietary propensities include:

- **Entire Foods:** Focus on entire, supplement thick food varieties, like organic products, vegetables, entire grains, lean proteins, and solid fats, to fuel your body with fundamental nutrients, minerals, and cell reinforcements.
- **Adjusted Macronutrients**: Keep a decent admission of sugars, proteins, and fats custom-made to your singular requirements and action levels. Balance macronutrients to help energy creation, muscle fix, and metabolic capability.
- **Hydration**: Remain satisfactorily hydrated by drinking water over the day. Hydration upholds cell hydration, supplement transport, detoxification cycles, and generally physiological capability.
- **Feast Planning:** Plan and get ready nutritious dinners and snacks ahead of time to limit hasty food decisions, save time, and advance consistency in dietary propensities. Integrate assortment, variety, and flavors to upgrade dinner satisfaction and healthful variety.

4. Physical Movement and Exercise

Customary actual work assumes an urgent part in enhancing cardiovascular well-being, strong strength, adaptability, and generally actual wellness. Integrate different activity modalities custom-fitted to your wellness level and objectives:

- ❖ **Cardiovascular Exercise:** Participate in high-impact exercises, like energetic strolling, running, cycling, or swimming, to work on cardiovascular perseverance, advance calorie use, and improve heart well-being.
- ❖ **Strength Training:** Coordinate opposition preparing works, like weightlifting, bodyweight activities, or

obstruction groups, to develop muscle fortitude, improve bone thickness, and back utilitarian development designs.

❖ **Adaptability and Mobility**: Consolidate extending, yoga, or portability activities to further develop adaptability, joint scope of movement, and postural arrangement. Adaptability preparing improves strong unwinding diminishes solidness, and supports injury avoidance.

❖ **Utilitarian Fitness:** Incorporate useful activities that impersonate day-to-day developments and exercises, like squats, rushes, or iron weight swings, to further develop equilibrium, coordination, and solid perseverance in genuine situations.

5. Sleep Cleanliness and Helpful Practices

Quality rest is fundamental for actual recuperation, mental capability, close-to-home prosperity, and general well-being. Focus on rest cleanliness practices and helpful exercises to help ideal rest quality and term:

- **Rest Schedule:** Lay out a predictable rest plan by heading to sleep and awakening simultaneously every day, even at the end of the week. Predictable rest designs control circadian rhythms and advance helpful rest cycles.

- **Rest Environment:** Establish a favorable rest climate that is dim, calm, and agreeable. Limit openness to electronic gadgets, screens, and invigorating exercises before sleep time to work with unwinding and plan for rest.

- **Unwinding Techniques**: Practice unwinding strategies, like moderate muscle unwinding, profound breathing activities, or directed symbolism, to advance actual unwinding, mental tranquility, and stress decrease before sleep time.

- **Computerized Detox:** Limit openness to electronic gadgets, cell phones, and screens at night hours to decrease blue light openness and invigorate melatonin creation. Make a breeze-down schedule that flags your body and psyche to progress from alertness to rest.

6. Stress the executives and Profound Resilience

Compelling pressure the executive's methodologies upgrade close to home strength, mental capability, and generally speaking prosperity during the Transformation venture. Investigate assorted ways to deal with alleviate pressure and cultivate close-to-home equilibrium:

- **Care Meditation:** Develop care through reflection rehearses that emphasize present-second mindfulness, acknowledgment, and non-critical perception of considerations and feelings.

- **Stress Decrease Techniques:** Integrate pressure-lessening exercises, like yoga, judo, moderate muscle unwinding, or nature strolls, to advance unwinding, lighten strain, and reestablish physiological equilibrium.

- **Mental Conduct Techniques:** Apply mental social procedures, like mental rebuilding, positive reevaluating, and critical thinking systems, to challenge negative idea designs, improve adapting abilities, and elevate versatile reactions to stressors.

- **Social Support:** Look for social help from companions, relatives, or care groups to share encounters, get consolation, and encourage a feeling of having a place and profound association during testing times.

7. Self-Care and Individual Well-being

Focus on taking care of oneself practices that sustain physical, mental, and close-to-home prosperity, advancing all-encompassing equilibrium and versatility all through your Transformation process:

- **Taking care of oneself Rituals:** Lay out taking care of oneself customs, for example, journaling, imaginative articulation, side interests, or spa medicines, to advance unwinding, self-reflection, and individual revival.

- **Time Management:** Oversee time successfully by focusing on assignments, defining limits, and apportioning devoted time for taking care of oneself exercises, side interests, and significant pursuits that advance individual satisfaction and life fulfillment.

- **Appreciation Practice:** Develop an appreciation practice by recognizing and valuing positive parts of your life, connections, and Transformation venture. Appreciation encourages close-to-home versatility, upgrades idealism, and advances generally speaking prosperity.

3.13 Pre-Transformation Detox Tips

Planning for a groundbreaking excursion includes something beyond defining objectives and get-together assets — it requires establishing areas of strength for a point for progress by enhancing your body and psyche. Detoxification, with regards to well-being and health, alludes to the most common way of wiping out poisons and debasements from the body to improve generally speaking prosperity and backing practical Transformation. This section investigates successful pre-Transformation detox tips to purge your body, restore your well-being, and launch your excursion toward lively living.

Figuring out Detoxification

Detoxification is a characteristic physiological cycle through which the body kills destructive substances, metabolic side effects, and ecological poisons. While the liver, kidneys, lungs, lymphatic framework, and skin are essential detoxification organs, supporting these frameworks through way-of-life adjustments and designated intercessions can advance detoxification pathways and advance all-encompassing well-being.

Advantages of Pre-Transformation Detox

Participating in a pre-Transformation detox routine offers various likely advantages, including:

- **Upgraded Supplement Absorption**: Purging the assemblage of poisons and enhancing gut-related capability might work on supplement ingestion and use, supporting general well-being and imperativeness.

- **Expanded Energy Levels**: Disposing of harmful weight and advancing detoxification pathways can upgrade energy levels, mental clearness, and actual endurance, working with commitment in groundbreaking exercises.

- **Further developed Metabolism:** Supporting liver capability and metabolic cycles through detoxification practices might improve metabolic productivity, work with weight the board, and back in general metabolic wellbeing.

- **Improved Insusceptible Function:** Detoxification upholds safe strength by lessening foundational aggravation, supporting cancer prevention agent protections, and advancing cell respectability.

- More clear Skin and Brilliant Complexion: Wiping out poisons and advancing lymphatic waste might further develop skin well-being, lessen imperfections, and upgrade skin brilliance during the Transformation interaction.

Pre-Transformation Detox Systems

Viable pre-Transformation detox techniques integrate comprehensive ways to deal with purging the body, support detoxification pathways, and enhance generally speaking prosperity. Consider incorporating these systems into your daily practice to set up your body and brain for a fruitful Transformation venture:

1. Nutrient-Thick Purging Diet

Embracing a supplement thick purging eating routine rich in entire food varieties, cell reinforcements, and phytonutrients can work with detoxification, sustain essential organs, and advance cell fix and recovery. Center around integrating:

1.**New Products of the soil:** Incorporate various bright leafy foods plentiful in nutrients, minerals, and cancer prevention agents to help detoxification pathways and improve cell wellbeing.

2.**Verdant Greens:** Consolidate mixed greens like kale, spinach, and arugula, which are plentiful in chlorophyll and backing liver detoxification processes.

3. **Cruciferous Vegetables:** Consume cruciferous vegetables like broccoli, Brussels fledglings, and cauliflower, which contain sulfur intensify and help stage II liver detoxification pathways.

4. **Berries:** Appreciate cancer prevention agent-rich berries like blueberries, strawberries, and raspberries, which assist with killing free revolutionaries, lessen oxidative pressure, and back cell honesty.

5. **Solid Fats**: Integrate sound fats from sources like avocado, nuts, seeds, and olive oil to help cell film respectability and work with fat-dissolvable poison end.

2. Hydration and Detoxifying Beverages

Hydration plays a vital part in supporting detoxification pathways, advancing kidney capability, and working with the disposal of metabolic byproducts and poisons from the body. Improve hydration and backing detoxification with:

a. **Water:** Drink a sufficient measure of sifted water over the day to help kidney capability, keep up with electrolyte balance, and work with poison disposal using pee.

b. Homegrown **Teas:** Appreciate detoxifying natural teas, for example, dandelion root tea, ginger tea, turmeric tea, and milk thorn tea, which support liver detoxification, advance bile creation, and help processing.

c. **Lemon Water**: Begin your day with warm lemon water to animate processing, alkalize the body, support liver capability, and improve bile creation for ideal detoxification.

d. **Detox Smoothies:** Get ready to supplement thick detox smoothies utilizing fixings, for example, salad greens, berries, avocado, coconut water, and chia seeds to help detoxification, advance satiety, and give fundamental supplements.

3. Elimination of Handled Food sources and Toxins

Limit openness to handled food sources, counterfeit added substances, additives, refined sugars, trans fats, and natural poisons that can trouble detoxification organs and hinder metabolic capability. Zero in on:

- **Entire Foods:** Pick natural, non-GMO entire food varieties at whatever point conceivable to lessen openness to pesticides, herbicides, and manufactured synthetics that might slow down detoxification pathways.

- **Sugar Reduction:** Cutoff utilization of refined sugars, sweet drinks, and handled tidbits, which add to Inflammation, insulin opposition, and metabolic unsettling influences.

- **Liquor and Caffeine Moderation**: Decrease liquor admission and moderate caffeine utilization to help liver capability, advance hydration, and limit oxidative pressure during the detoxification interaction.

- **Aversion of Ecological Toxins**: Limit openness to natural poisons tracked down in family cleaners, individual consideration items, plastics, and contaminations that can gather in the body and disturb detoxification pathways.

4. Enhanced Liver Support

The liver assumes a focal part in detoxification by utilizing poisons, blending bile acids, and working with the end side effects of the body. Support liver well-being and upgrade detoxification pathways with:

- **Liver-Purging Foods:** Remember food sources rich in liver-purifying supplements like sulfur (e.g., garlic, onions), cell reinforcements (e.g., berries, mixed greens), and amino acids (e.g., lean proteins) to help stage I and stage II liver detoxification pathways.

- **Milk Thistle:** Consider enhancing with milk thorn, a plant spice known for its hepatoprotective properties and capacity to help liver capability, advance bile creation, and work with poison end.

- **Cruciferous Vegetables**: Integrate cruciferous vegetables, for example, broccoli, Brussels fledglings, and cabbage, which contain glucosinolates and sulfur that help liver detoxification processes.

- **Hydration:** Hydrate and natural teas to help kidney capability, advance pee creation, and work with the disposal of water-dissolvable poisons and metabolic byproducts.

5. Promotion of Lymphatic Drainage

The lymphatic framework assumes a fundamental part in safe capability, liquid equilibrium, and the evacuation of cell byproducts and poisons from the body. Support lymphatic seepage and flow with:

a. **Dry Brushing:** Integrate dry brushing methods utilizing a characteristic fiber brush to invigorate lymphatic dissemination, further develop complexion, and advance the end of metabolic side-effects through lymphatic vessels.

b. Practice **and Movement:** Take part in standard actual work, like yoga, bouncing back, energetic strolling, or swimming, to advance lymphatic dissemination, improve liquid elements, and back poison disposal.

c. **Rub Therapy:** Consider lymphatic waste back rub procedures performed by a certified specialist to invigorate lymphatic course, decrease liquid maintenance, and back detoxification processes.

d. **Hydration:** Hydrate over the day to keep up with hydration, support kidney capability, and work with the end of metabolic byproducts and poisons using pee and lymphatic seepage.

6. Mind-Body Practices for Pressure Reduction

Stress decrease methods assume a significant part in supporting detoxification pathways, advancing close-to-home prosperity, and improving by and large well-being during the Transformation cycle. Consolidate mind-body practices, for example,

a. **Profound Breathing Exercises:** Practice profound breathing activities, diaphragmatic breathing, or pranayama procedures to advance unwinding, decrease pressure chemicals, and backing detoxification.

b. **Reflection and Mindfulness**: Participate in care contemplation practices to develop present-second mindfulness, improve pressure strength, and advance profound equilibrium during the detoxification cycle.

c. **Yoga and Stretching:** Integrate yoga presents, delicate extending activities, or helpful yoga practices to deliver pressure, further develop adaptability, and backing detoxification through improved flow and lymphatic seepage.

CHAPTER 4: The 7-Day Plan Outline

Changing your body and well-being in only multi week requires an extensive, balanced approach that incorporates dietary Transformations as well as workout schedules and care rehearses. This section gives a point-by-point step-by-step breakdown, everyday feast plans, workout schedules, and care and stress decrease strategies to assist you with accomplishing your objectives of cooling Inflammation, recuperating your gut, and changing your general prosperity.

4.11 Step by step Breakdown

The 7-Day Plan is organized to slowly acquaint you with new propensities and schedules that will uphold your well-being and health venture. Every day expands on the past one, guaranteeing a comprehensive way to deal with Transformation.

Day 1: Detox and Rejuvenate - Center on detoxifying your body and setting it up for the week ahead.

Day 2: Gut Wellbeing Focus - Focus on gut well-being with probiotic-rich food varieties and delicate gut-related help.

Day 3: Cancer prevention agent Boost - Integrate cell reinforcement-rich food sources to battle Inflammation and oxidative pressure.

Day 4: Strength and Flexibility - Participate in exercises that develop fortitude and upgrade adaptability.

Day 5: Psyche Body Connection - Underline the association between actual well-being and mental prosperity.

Day 6: Revival and Recovery - Permit your body to recuperate and restore with delicate exercises and sustaining food sources.

Day 7: Reflect and Celebrate - Ponder your advancement and praise your accomplishments with a decent, compensating day.

4.12 Day- to- day Feast Plans

Every day's feast plan is intended to be adjusted, supported, and simple to follow. Here is an outline of the everyday feast structure:

Day 1: Detox and Rejuvenate

- Breakfast: Green Smoothie (spinach, kale, avocado, chia seeds, almond milk, plant-based protein powder)

- Early in the day Snack: New natural product (apple or berries)

- Lunch: Rainbow Salad (blended greens, cherry tomatoes, cucumbers, ringer peppers, quinoa, lemon-tahini dressing, barbecued chicken or chickpeas)

- Evening Snack: Nuts and seeds

- Dinner: Heated Salmon (turmeric and ginger flavoring) with steamed broccoli and yams

- Evening Snack: Carrot sticks and hummus

Day 2: Gut Wellbeing Focus

- Breakfast: Probiotic Smoothie Bowl (kefir, banana, spinach, granola, chia seeds)
- Early in the day Snack: Greek yogurt with honey and flaxseeds
- Lunch: Vegetable Soup (bone stock, carrots, celery, kale, lentils)
- Evening Snack: Aged vegetables (kimchi or sauerkraut)

- Dinner: Aged food plate (barbecued vegetables, quinoa, kimchi or sauerkraut)
- Evening Snack: Ginger tea

Day 3: Cancer prevention agent Boost

✓ Breakfast: Cancer prevention agent Smoothie Bowl (açai, blueberries, spinach, almond margarine, coconut drops, hemp seeds)
✓ Early in the day Snack: New berries (blueberries or strawberries)
✓ Lunch: Rainbow Salad (blended greens, broiled beets, carrots, chime peppers, avocado, citrus vinaigrette, barbecued shrimp or chickpeas)
✓ Evening Snack: Green tea
✓ Dinner: Broiled Vegetables with Quinoa (wild-got salmon or marinated tofu, rosemary, thyme)
✓ Evening Snack: Dull chocolate (little piece, 70% cacao or higher)

Day 4: Strength and Flexibility

- Breakfast: Green Smoothie (spinach, kale, banana, almond milk, protein powder)

- Early in the day Snack: Oats Bowl (new berries, nuts, seeds)

- Lunch: Barbecued Chicken Plate of mixed greens (blended greens, barbecued chicken or tofu, broiled Brussels sprouts, quinoa salad)

- Evening Snack: Nuts and seeds

- Dinner: Vegetable Pan fried food (earthy colored rice or cauliflower rice, vivid vegetables, lean protein)

- Evening Snack: Chamomile tea

Day 5: Brain-Body Connection

1. Breakfast: Smoothie (blended berries, spinach, chia seeds, almond milk)

2. Early in the day Snack: Natural tea (chamomile or lavender)

3. Lunch: Buddha Bowl (blended greens, cooked yams, chickpeas, avocado, tahini dressing)

4. Evening Snack: Green tea

5. Dinner: Barbecued Fish or Tempeh (steamed asparagus, wild rice)

6. Evening Snack: Peppermint tea

Day 6: Revival and Recovery

- Breakfast: Green Juice (celery, cucumber, green apple, parsley)
- Early in the day Snack: Protein Smoothie Bowl (Greek yogurt, new organic product, nuts, seeds)
- Lunch: Sustaining Salad (blended greens, barbecued chicken or tofu, simmered vegetables, balsamic vinaigrette)
- Evening Snack: Home-grown tea (dandelion tea)
- Dinner: Vegetable Curry (lentils, earthy colored rice, vegetables, turmeric, cumin)
- Evening Snack: Ginger tea

Day 7: Reflect and Celebrate

- Breakfast: Supplement Thick Smoothie (blended berries, spinach, chia seeds, almond milk)

- Early in the day Snack: New natural product (apple or berries)

- Lunch: Adjusted Feast (barbecued salmon or tofu, simmered vegetables, quinoa)

- Evening Snack: Green tea

- Dinner: Celebratory Feast (healthy, supplement thick elements of your decision)

- Evening Snack: Chamomile tea

4.13 Work-out Schedules

Standard actual work is significant for diminishing Inflammation, further developing gut well-being, and supporting general prosperity. Here is a breakdown of work-out schedules for every day:

Day 1: Moderate Cardio

- 30 minutes of lively strolling or cycling to help course and advance detoxification.

Day 2: Delicate Yoga

- 30-minute yoga meeting zeroing in on delicate stretches and represents advanced assimilation and unwinding.

Day 3: HIIT Session

- 30-minute stop-and-go aerobic exercise (HIIT) to help digestion and upgrade cardiovascular well-being.

Day 4: Strength Training

- 30-minute strength instructional course focusing on significant muscle gatherings to develop fortitude and further develop adaptability.

Day 5: Pilates

- 30-minute Pilates meeting to reinforce your center and further develop body arrangement.

Day 6: Helpful Walk

- Delicate, helpful stroll in nature to associate with your environmental factors and advance unwinding.

Day 7: Delicate Yoga

- 30-minute yoga meeting zeroing in on delicate stretches and unwinding to ponder your advancement and praise your accomplishments.

4.14 Care and Stress Decrease Strategies

Mental and profound prosperity are vital to your Transformation process. Every day, consolidate care and stress decrease methods to help a fair psyche-body association:

Morning Meditation:

- Begin every day with a 10-brief care contemplation zeroing in on appreciation, breath mindfulness, and setting positive expectations.

Noontime Mindfulness:

- Require a couple of moments during lunch to rehearse careful eating, focusing on the flavors, surfaces, and vibes of your food.

Evening Relaxation:

- Wind down each night with a quieting movement, for example, journaling, perusing, or paying attention to mitigating music. Consider your day, noticing any sure Transformations or progress.

Breathing Exercises:

- Consolidate profound breathing activities over the day to lessen pressure and advance unwinding. Practice diaphragmatic breathing or the 4-7-8 breathing method.

Moderate Muscle Relaxation:

- Take part in moderate muscle unwinding activities to deliver strain and advance physical and mental unwinding.

Day 1: Launching Your Transformation

Welcome to Day 1 of your Transformation process! This first day establishes the vibe for the week ahead, zeroing in on supporting your body with mitigating food varieties, taking part in delicate activity, and rehearsing care strategies to diminish pressure and advance in general prosperity. Toward the finish of today, you will have moved toward cooling Inflammation, recuperating your gut, and setting areas of strength for enduring well-being and imperativeness.

Breakfast: Mitigating Smoothie

Begin your day with a supplement pressed Mitigating Smoothie. This scrumptious mix tastes perfect as well as intended to battle aggravation and furnishes your body with fundamental nutrients and minerals.

Ingredients:

- 1 cup spinach

- 1 cup kale

- 1/2 avocado

- 1 tablespoon chia seeds

- 1 cup unsweetened almond milk

- 1/2 cup frozen berries (blueberries, strawberries, or raspberries)

- 1 scoop plant-based protein powder

- 1 teaspoon turmeric

- 1 teaspoon ginger

Instructions:

1. Add all fixings to a high-velocity blender.

2. Mix until smooth and rich.

3. Fill a glass and appreciate right away.

Benefits:

- Spinach and Kale: Loaded with cancer prevention agents and mitigating compounds.

- Avocado: Gives sound fats and a velvety surface.

- Chia Seeds: Wealthy in omega-3 unsaturated fats, which assist with decreasing Inflammation.

- Berries: High in cancer prevention agents, which battle oxidative pressure.

- Turmeric and Ginger: Known for their powerful calming properties.

This smoothie will pass you feeling stimulated and prepared to require on the day, giving a strong beginning to your Transformation process.

Lunch: Gut Mending Salad

For lunch, partake in a Gut Mending Salad that is both fulfilling and valuable for your gut-related well-being. This salad is rich in fiber, prebiotics, and probiotics, which assist with supporting a sound gut microbiome.

Ingredients:

- Leafy greens (spinach, arugula, and kale)

- 1/2 cup cooked quinoa

- 1/2 cup destroyed carrots

- 1/2 cup cut cucumbers

- 1/2 cup cherry tomatoes split

- 1/4 cup aged vegetables (kimchi or sauerkraut)

- 1/4 cup chickpeas or barbecued chicken for protein

- 1/4 avocado, cut

- Lemon-tahini dressing (1 tablespoon tahini, juice of 1 lemon, 1 tablespoon olive oil, salt, and pepper to taste)

Instructions:

1. Join blended greens, quinoa, carrots, cucumbers, cherry tomatoes, and matured vegetables in an enormous bowl.

2. Top with chickpeas or barbecued chicken and avocado cuts.

3. Shower with lemon-tahini dressing and throw to consolidate.

Benefits:

- Blended Greens: Give various nutrients and minerals.

- Quinoa: A total protein and high in fiber.

- Aged Vegetables: Wealthy in probiotics, which backs gut wellbeing.

- Chickpeas/Barbecued Chicken: Offers a decent wellspring of protein.

- Avocado: Adds solid fats and smoothness.

This salad is an ideal late-morning dinner that upholds processing, advances gut well-being, and keeps you full and stimulated over the evening.

Supper: Lean Protein with Veggies

End your day with a reasonable supper of Lean Protein with Veggies. This dinner is intended to be light yet fulfilling, helping your body recuperate and get ready for the following day.

Ingredients:

- 1 serving of lean protein (salmon, chicken bosom, or tofu)

- 1 cup broccoli florets

- 1 cup cut chime peppers

- 1 cup cherry tomatoes

- 1 tablespoon olive oil

- Salt, pepper, and your number one spices (rosemary, thyme, or oregano)

Instructions:

1. Preheat your broiler to 375°F (190c)

2. Put the rest protein on a baking sheet and season with salt, pepper, and spices.

3. Organize the broccoli, chime peppers, and cherry tomatoes around the protein, shower with olive oil, and season with extra spices.

4. Heat for 20-25 minutes or until the protein is cooked through and the vegetables are delicate.

5. Serve right away.

Benefits:

- Fit Protein: Fundamental for muscle fix and development.

- Broccoli: High in fiber and nutrients.

- Ringer Peppers: Plentiful in cancer prevention agents and L-ascorbic acid.

- Cherry Tomatoes: Give lycopene, a cancer prevention agent with mitigating properties.

This feast guarantees you end your day with a nutritious, calming supper that upholds your body's recuperating processes.

Work out Delicate Yoga

Integrating delicate yoga into your everyday schedule diminishes pressure, further, develops adaptability, and advances generally speaking prosperity. The present yoga meeting will zero in on delicate stretches and represent improved processing and unwinding.

Routine:

1. Child's Posture (Balasana): Start in a stooping position, sit out of sorts, and broaden your arms forward, laying your brow on the mat. Hold for 2-3 minutes.

2. Cat-Cow Stretch (Marjaryasana-Bitilasana): On all fours, shift back and forth between curving your back (Cow) and adjusting it (Feline). Rehash for 5-10 breaths.

3. Seated Forward Twist (Paschimottanasana): Sit with your legs expanded, reach forward, and hold your feet or shins. Hold for 2-3 minutes.

4. Supine Turn (Supta Matsyendrasana): Lie on your back, carry your knees to your chest, and delicately lower them aside. Hold for 1-2 minutes on each side.

5. Corpse Posture (Savasana): Untruth level on your back, arms at your sides, and shut your eyes. Center around your breath and unwind for 5-10 minutes.

Benefits:

- Diminishes Stress: Advances unwinding and decreases cortisol levels.

- Further develops Digestion: Invigorates the gut-related organs and further develops gut wellbeing.

- Upgrades Flexibility: Tenderly stretches and protracts muscles.

Care: Profound Breathing Activities

Rehearsing profound breathing activities can fundamentally diminish pressure and advance a feeling of quiet and prosperity. These activities are basic, should be possible anyplace, and are especially viable when integrated into your everyday daily schedule.

Work out: 4-7-8 breathing

1. Sit or rest in an agreeable position.

2. Shut your eyes and take a full breath through your nose for a count of 4.

3. Pause your breathing for a count of 7.

4. Breathe out leisurely through your mouth for a count of 8.

5. Rehash this cycle 4-5 times.

Benefits:

- Diminishes Stress: Enacts the parasympathetic sensory system, advancing unwinding.

- Further develops Focus: Increments oxygen stream to the mind, improving fixation.

- Balances Emotions: Oversees tension and advances close to home steadiness.

Work out: Diaphragmatic Breathing

1. Sit or rest easily with one hand on your chest and the other on your mid-region.

2. Take a sluggish, full breath in through your nose, permitting your gut (not your chest) to grow.

3. Breathe out leisurely through your mouth.

4. Center around the ascent and fall of your mid-region. Rehash for 5-10 minutes.

Benefits:

- Upgrades Relaxation: Advances an underground government of quiet.

- Further develops Lung Function: Fortifies the gut and improves respiratory proficiency.

- Brings down Blood Pressure: Decreases pressure prompted hypertension.

Day 2: Supporting Your Digestion

Welcome to Day 2 of your extraordinary excursion! The present spotlight is on helping your digestion to help your body's innate capacity to consume calories and keep up with energy levels. By consolidating supplement thick dinners wealthy in omega-3 unsaturated fats, probiotics, and mitigating fixings, close by a strengthening cardio meeting and care practice, you'll make way for supported metabolic well-being and by and large prosperity.

Breakfast: Omega-3 Rich Breakfast Bowl

Launch your digestion with a delightful Omega-3 Rich Breakfast Bowl. This breakfast is loaded with sound fats, fiber, and protein, guaranteeing you starts your day with supported energy and a metabolic lift.

Ingredients:

- 1/2 cup moved oats

- 1 cup unsweetened almond milk

- 1 tablespoon chia seeds

- 1 tablespoon flaxseeds

- 1/2 cup blended berries (blueberries, strawberries, raspberries)

- 1/4 avocado, diced

- 1 tablespoon almond margarine

- 1 teaspoon honey (discretionary)

Instructions:

1. In a bowl, join moved oats and almond milk. Allow it to sit for a couple of moments to mellow or microwave for 1-2 minutes.

2. Mix in chia seeds and flaxseeds.

3. Top with blended berries, avocado, and almond spread.

4. Shower with honey whenever wanted.

Benefits:

- Oats: Give complex carbs and fiber to support energy.

- Chia and Flaxseeds: Wealthy in omega-3 unsaturated fats that help heart wellbeing and decrease Inflammation.

- Berries: High in cancer prevention agents and nutrients.

- Avocado: Offers sound fats that advance satiety and back digestion.

- Almond Butter: Adds protein and sound fats.

This morning meal bowl fills your body as well as keeps up with stable glucose levels, forestalling early-in-the-day energy crashes and keeping your digestion dynamic.

Lunch: Aged Food sources Gala

For lunch, enjoy a Matured Food Sources Gala that supports gut wellbeing and digestion. Matured food sources are rich in probiotics, which assist with adjusting your gut microbiome and improve supplement assimilation.

Ingredients:

- Leafy greens (spinach, arugula, and kale)

- 1/2 cup quinoa

- 1/2 cup destroyed carrots

- 1/2 cup cut cucumbers

- 1/4 cup matured vegetables (kimchi or sauerkraut)

- 1/4 cup edamame

- 1/4 avocado, cut

- 1/4 cup salted red onions

- Lemon-ginger dressing (1 tablespoon olive oil, juice of 1 lemon, 1 teaspoon ground ginger, salt, and pepper to taste)

Instructions:

1. Consolidate blended greens, quinoa, carrots, cucumbers, matured vegetables, edamame, and avocado in a huge bowl.

2. Top with cured red onions.

3. Shower with lemon-ginger dressing and throw to consolidate.

Benefits:

- Aged Vegetables: Give probiotics that help gut wellbeing.

- Edamame: Offers plant-based protein and fiber.

- Salted Red Onions: Add flavor and probiotics.

- Lemon-Ginger Dressing: Upgrades assimilation and has calming properties.

This lunch upholds a solid gut as well as lifts your digestion, as a reasonable gut microbiome is fundamental for effective metabolic capability.

Supper: Calming Soup

End your day with a warming bowl of Calming Soup. This supper is light yet fulfilling, loaded with fixings known for their calming and digestion-supporting properties.

Ingredients:

- 1 tablespoon olive oil

- 1 onion, slashed

- 2 garlic cloves, minced

- 1-inch piece of ginger, ground

- 1 teaspoon turmeric

- 1 teaspoon cumin

- 1 cup diced carrots

- 1 cup diced celery

- 1 cup slashed kale

- 1 can (14.5 oz) diced tomatoes

- 4 cups vegetable stock

- 1 cup cooked chickpeas

- Salt and pepper to taste

- New cilantro for embellish

Instructions:

1. Heat olive oil in a huge pot over medium intensity. Add onion, garlic, and ginger, and sauté until fragrant.

2. Add turmeric and cumin, mixing to join.

3. Add carrots, celery, and kale, and cook for a couple of moments.

4. Pour in diced tomatoes and vegetable stock. Heat to the point of boiling, then, at that point, decrease to a stew.

5. Add chickpeas and stew for 15-20 minutes until vegetables are delicate.

6. Season with salt and pepper.

7. Decorate with new cilantro before serving.

Benefits:

- Turmeric and Ginger: Strong calming properties.

- Vegetables: Give fiber, nutrients, and minerals.

- Chickpeas: Offer plant-based protein and fiber.

This soup alleviates your gut-related framework as well as lessens aggravation, advancing by and large metabolic well-being.

Work out: Cardio Meeting

A vital part of helping your digestion is consolidating standard cardiovascular activity. The present cardio meeting will assist with expanding your pulse, consuming calories, and improving metabolic effectiveness.

Routine:

1. Warm-Up: 5-10 minutes of light running or lively strolling to set up your body.

2. High-Force Span Preparing (HIIT):

   - Hopping Jacks: 1 moment

   - Burpees: 1 moment

   - Mountain Climbers: 1 moment

   - High Knees: 1 moment

   - Rest: 1 moment

   - Rehash the circuit 3-4 times.

3. Cool-Down: 5-10 minutes of slow strolling and extending to cut your pulse down bit by bit.

Benefits:

- Consumes Calories: Assists with the weight of the board and supporting digestion.

- Works on Cardiovascular Health: Fortifies your heart and lungs.

- Upgrades Metabolic Rate: Builds your body's capacity to productively consume calories.

Care: Directed Reflection

End your day with a Directed Reflection to quiet your brain, lessen pressure, and advance a feeling of harmony and prosperity. Care rehearses are critical for overseeing feelings of anxiety, which can influence metabolic well-being.

Exercise:

1. Track down a peaceful, agreeable spot to sit or rest.

2. Shut your eyes and take a couple of full breaths, zeroing in on the vibe of the air entering and leaving your body.

3. Follow this directed reflection script:

- "Start by focusing on your breath. Notice the normal beat of your relaxing. There is a compelling reason to transform it; simply notice.
- As you keep on breathing, envision a warm, quieting light entering your body with each breath in. This light brings harmony and unwinding.
- With each breath out, discharge any pressure or stress, permitting your body to sink further into unwinding.
- Presently, carry your attention to your body. Begin at your toes and gradually check upwards, seeing any areas of pressure or uneasiness. As you distinguish these regions, envision the warm light alleviating and loosening up them.
- Proceed with this cycle until you have checked the whole body.
- At the point when you are prepared, tenderly take your mindfulness back to your breath. Take a couple of additional full breaths, and when you feel prepared, gradually open your eyes."

Benefits:

- Decreases Stress: Brings down cortisol levels, which can influence digestion.

- Advances Relaxation: Improves general mental prosperity.

- Further develops Focus: Helps clear the brain and further develop fixation.

Day 3: Recuperating Your Gut

Welcome to Day 3 of your Transformation process! The present spotlight is on recuperating your gut, a fundamental stage in advancing general well-being and prosperity. A sound gut upholds processing as well as impacts your resistant framework, state of mind, and energy levels. By consolidating probiotic-rich food varieties, fiber, and incline proteins toward your feasts, alongside strength preparation and care journaling, you'll establish a climate where your gut can flourish.

Breakfast: Probiotic Yogurt Parfait

Begin your day with a scrumptious and supporting Probiotic Yogurt Parfait. This morning meal is intended to furnish your body with gainful microscopic organisms, fundamental supplements, and energy to fuel your morning exercises.

Ingredients:

- 1 cup plain Greek yogurt (or a sans dairy elective with live societies)

- 1/2 cup granola (ideally low-sugar and high-fiber)

- 1/2 cup blended berries (blueberries, strawberries, raspberries)

- 1 tablespoon honey or maple syrup (discretionary)

- 1 tablespoon chia seeds

- 1 tablespoon flaxseeds

Instructions:

1. Spoon half of the Greek yogurt into a bowl or glass.

2. Layer with half of the granola and blended berries.

3. Add the leftover yogurt, trailed by the remainder of the granola and berries.

4. Shower with honey or maple syrup whenever wanted.

5. Sprinkle chia seeds and flaxseeds on top for added fiber and omega-3 unsaturated fats.

Benefits:

- Greek Yogurt: Wealthy in probiotics that help a sound gut microbiome.

- Granola: Gives fiber and complex sugars to support energy.

- Berries: High in cell reinforcements and nutrients.

- Chia and Flaxseeds: Offer omega-3 unsaturated fats and fiber.

This yogurt parfait is a heavenly and simple method for integrating probiotics and fiber into your eating routine, supporting gut-related well-being and giving an explosion of energy to begin your day.

Lunch: Entire Grain Wraps

For lunch, appreciate nutritious and fulfilling Entire Grain Wraps. These wraps are loaded with fiber-rich fixings and lean protein, supporting gut well-being and giving supported energy over the day.

Ingredients:

- Entire grain tortillas or wraps

- 1/2 cup hummus

- 1/2 cup destroyed carrots

- 1/2 cup cut cucumbers

- 1/2 cup child spinach leaves

- 1/4 cup cut chime peppers

- 1/4 cup disintegrated feta cheddar (discretionary)

- 1/4 cup cooked quinoa or earthy-colored rice

- 1/4 avocado, cut

- Lemon-tahini dressing (1 tablespoon tahini, juice of 1 lemon, 1 tablespoon olive oil, salt, and pepper to taste)

Instructions:

1. Spread hummus equitably over the entire grain tortillas.

2. Layer with destroyed carrots, cucumbers, spinach, ringer peppers, and quinoa or earthy-colored rice.

3. Add disintegrated feta cheddar if utilizing, and top with avocado cuts.

4. Sprinkle with lemon-tahini dressing and roll up the tortillas to shape wraps.

Benefits:

- Entire Grain Tortillas: High in fiber, which upholds gut-related well-being.

- Hummus: Produced using chickpeas, giving fiber and protein.

- Vegetables: Offer nutrients, minerals, and cancer prevention agents.

- Quinoa/Brown Rice: Adds complex starches and extra fiber.

These wraps are delightful as well as loaded with supplements that advance gut well-being, making them a great decision for a noontime dinner.

Supper: Fish and Veggie Pan fried food

End your day with a light yet fulfilling Fish and Veggie Pan fried food. This supper is rich in lean protein, solid fats, and different vegetables, all of which add to a sound gut.

Ingredients:

- 1 tablespoon olive oil

- 1 garlic clove, minced

- 1-inch piece of ginger, ground

- 1 cup broccoli florets

- 1 cup cut chime peppers

- 1 cup snap peas

- 1/2 cup cut mushrooms

- 1 filet of fish (like salmon or cod), cut into scaled-down pieces

- 2 tablespoons low-sodium soy sauce or tamari

- 1 tablespoon rice vinegar

- 1 teaspoon honey or maple syrup

- 1/4 cup hacked green onions

- Cooked earthy-colored rice or quinoa for serving

Instructions:

1. Heat olive oil in a huge skillet or wok over medium-high intensity. Add garlic and ginger, and sauté until fragrant.

2. Add broccoli, chime peppers, snap peas, and mushrooms. Pan-sear for 5-7 minutes until vegetables are delicate and fresh.

3. Push the vegetables to the side of the skillet and add the fish pieces. Cook for 2-3 minutes on each side until cooked through.

4. Consolidate soy sauce, rice vinegar, and honey in a little bowl. Pour over the fish and vegetables, mixing to equally cover.

5. Eliminate from intensity and sprinkle with cleaved green onions.

6. Serve over cooked earthy-colored rice or quinoa.

Benefits:

- Fish: Gives lean protein and omega-3 unsaturated fats.

- Vegetables: Plentiful in fiber, nutrients, and minerals.

- Olive Oil: Offers sound fats that help heart wellbeing.

This pan-fried food isn't just tasty but additionally loaded with supplements that advance gut well-being and general prosperity.

Work out: Strength Preparing

Integrating strength preparation into your routine is fundamental for building muscle, helping digestion, and supporting general well-being. The present strength instructional meeting centers on significant muscle gatherings and advances metabolic well-being.

Routine:

1. Warm-Up: 5-10 minutes of light cardio, like lively strolling or running.

2. Strength Preparing Circuit:

   - Squats: 3 arrangements of 12 reps

   - Push-Ups: 3 arrangements of 10 reps

   - Free weight Rows: 3 arrangements of 12 reps for every side

   - Lunges: 3 arrangements of 12 reps for each side

   - Plank: Hold for 1 moment

3. Cool-Down: 5-10 minutes of extending, zeroing in on the muscles worked.

Benefits:

- Constructs Muscle: Increments bulk, which helps digestion.

- Further develops Strength: Improves in general actual strength and perseverance.

- Upholds Metabolism: Muscle tissue consumes a larger number of calories very still than fat tissue.

Care: Journaling

End your day with a care practice that advances self-reflection and profound prosperity. Journaling is an astounding method for handling your considerations, setting aims, and diminishing pressure.

Work out: Intelligent Journaling

1. Track down a calm, agreeable spot to sit with your diary and a pen.

2. Consider your day and expound on your encounters, zeroing in on the accompanying prompts:

  - What went well today?

  - What difficulties did you face?

  - How could you feel over the day?

  - What are you appreciative for today?

  - What are your expectations for tomorrow?

Benefits:

- Diminishes Stress: Helps process feelings and decrease uneasiness.

- Advances Self-Awareness: Energizes self-reflection and care.

- Improves Well-Being: Encourages a positive outlook and appreciation.

Day 4: Lessening Aggravation

Welcome to Day 4 of your extraordinary excursion! The present spotlight is on diminishing Inflammation, a key stage in advancing generally speaking well-being and forestalling persistent sicknesses. Aggravation, when persistent, can prompt different medical problems, including coronary illness, diabetes, and immune system conditions. By integrating calming food varieties, delicate yet successful activity, and care rehearses into your everyday daily schedule, you'll uphold your body's normal recuperating cycles and improve your general prosperity.

Breakfast: Turmeric and Ginger Tea

Begin your day with a calming and mending Turmeric and Ginger Tea. This drink is loaded with calming properties that can assist with decreasing Inflammation and backing generally speaking well-being.

Ingredients:

- 1 cup boiling water

- 1 teaspoon ground turmeric

- 1 teaspoon ground new ginger or 1/2 teaspoon ground ginger

- 1 tablespoon lemon juice

- 1 teaspoon honey or maple syrup (discretionary)

- A spot of dark pepper (to improve the ingestion of curcumin from turmeric)

Instructions:

1. Bubble water and let it cool somewhat.

2. Add turmeric and ginger to the boiling water.

3. Mix in lemon squeeze and honey or maple syrup if utilizing.

4. Add a touch of dark pepper.

5. Allow the tea to soak for 5-10 minutes before drinking.

Benefits:

- Turmeric: Contains curcumin, an intense mitigating compound.

- Ginger: Known for its calming and cell reinforcement properties.

- Lemon Juice: Gives L-ascorbic acid and cell reinforcements.

- Honey/Maple Syrup: Adds a hint of normal pleasantness and extra cell reinforcements.

This tea assists with diminishing Inflammation as well as fills in as a warm, encouraging method for beginning your day.

Lunch: Mitigating Power Bowl

For lunch, partake in a supplement thick Mitigating Power Bowl. This feast consolidates different calming fixings to make a heavenly and fulfilling dish that upholds your well-being and energy levels.

Ingredients:

- 1/2 cup cooked quinoa

- 1/2 cup chickpeas, depleted and washed

- 1/2 cup steamed broccoli

- 1/4 cup destroyed carrots

- 1/4 avocado, cut

- 1/4 cup pomegranate seeds

- 1 tablespoon chia seeds

- Small bunch of leafy greens (spinach, arugula, kale)

- Turmeric-tahini dressing (1 tablespoon tahini, 1 teaspoon turmeric, juice of 1 lemon, 1 tablespoon olive oil, salt, and pepper to taste)

Instructions:

1. Collect the blended greens at the foundation of your bowl.

2. Add cooked quinoa, chickpeas, steamed broccoli, destroyed carrots, avocado cuts, and pomegranate seeds on top.

3. Sprinkle with chia seeds.

4. Shower with turmeric-tahini dressing and throw to consolidate.

Benefits:

- Quinoa: Gives total protein and fiber.

- Chickpeas: Wealthy in protein and fiber, advancing satiety.

- Broccoli: High in nutrients, minerals, and cancer prevention agents.

- Pomegranate Seeds: Loaded with cell reinforcements and against inflammatory response.

Turmeric-Tahini Dressing: Adds flavor and further mitigating benefits.

This power bowl isn't just beautiful and appealing yet addition stacked with fixings that battle aggravation and feed your body.

Supper: Quinoa and Veggie Skillet

End your day with a good and tasty Quinoa and Veggie Skillet. This supper is loaded with vegetables, quinoa, and spices that give mitigating advantages and fundamental supplements.

Ingredients:

- 1 tablespoon olive oil

- 1 onion, hacked

- 2 garlic cloves, minced

- 1 red chime pepper, hacked

- 1 zucchini, hacked

- 1 cup cherry tomatoes, split

- 1 cup cooked quinoa

- 1 cup spinach leaves

- 1 teaspoon dried oregano

- 1 teaspoon dried basil

- Salt and pepper to taste

- New parsley for decorating

Instructions:

1. Heat olive oil in an enormous skillet over medium intensity. Add onion and garlic, and sauté until fragrant.

2. Add red chime pepper and zucchini, and cook until delicate.

3. Mix in cherry tomatoes and cook for a couple of additional minutes until they begin to mellow.

4. Add cooked quinoa, spinach, oregano, basil, salt, and pepper. Mix to consolidate and cook until the spinach withers.

5. Decorate with new parsley before serving.

Benefits:

- Quinoa: Gives total protein and fiber.

- Vegetables: Plentiful in nutrients, minerals, and cell reinforcements.

- Olive Oil: Contains sound fats and calming properties.

- Herbs: Oregano and basil add flavor and extra cell reinforcements.

This skillet dish is not difficult to get ready and overflowing with flavors and supplements that assist with lessening Inflammation and backing by and large well-being.

Work out Pilates

Pilates is a phenomenal activity decision for diminishing Inflammation. This low-influence exercise centers around center strength, adaptability, and general body arrangement, which can assist with lessening pressure and advance a fair, solid body.

Routine:

1. Warm-Up: 5-10 minutes of delicate extending to set up your body.

2. Pilates Exercises:

- ❖ Hundred: Lie on your back with your knees bowed at 90 degrees. Lift your head, neck, and shoulders off the mat, expanding your arms straight out. Siphon your arms all over for 100 counts, taking in for 5 excludes and for 5 counts.
- ❖ Roll-Up: Lie on your back with your legs straight and arms expanded above. Breathe in, lift your arms and head off the mat, and breathe out as you roll up to arrive at your toes. Breathe in to turn around the development, breathing out as you roll down.
- ❖ Single-Leg Stretch: Lie on your back with your knees twisted. Lift your head, neck, and shoulders off the mat, and expand your right leg while holding your left knee. Switch legs, pulling the contrary knee toward your chest.
- ❖ Twofold Leg Stretch: Lie on your back with your knees bowed and hands on your shins. Lift your head, neck, and shoulders off the mat, expanding your arms and legs all the while. Circle your arms and step your knees back to the beginning position.
- ❖ Plank: Start on all fours. Broaden your legs back, keeping your body in an orderly fashion from head to heels. Hold for 30-60 seconds, drawing in your center.

3. Cool-Down: 5-10 minutes of extending to loosen up your

Muscles.

Benefits:

- Center Strength: Constructs serious areas of strength for a center.

- Flexibility: Upgrades, by and large adaptability and decreases muscle solidness.

- Stress Reduction: Advances unwinding and lessens pressure.

Care: Perception Methods

End your day with a care practice that consolidates representation procedures. Representation can assist with lessening pressure, advancing unwinding, and upgrading your, generally speaking, mental prosperity.

Work out: Directed Visualization

1. Track down a tranquil, agreeable spot to sit or rest.

2. Shut your eyes and take a couple of full breaths, zeroing in on the vibe of the air entering and leaving your body.

3. Picture a tranquil, quiet place where you have a good sense of security and loss. This could be an ocean side, a woodland, or any spot that presents to you a feeling of quietness.

4. Envision yourself here, completely encountering it with every one of your faculties. Experience the glow of the sun, hear the delicate sound of waves or stirring leaves, and smell the outside air.

5. As you keep on breathing profoundly, envision any strain or stress liquefying ceaselessly. Feel your body becoming lighter and more loose with every breath.

6. Put shortly in this quiet spot, permitting yourself to drench in the experience completely.

7. At the point when you are prepared, delicately take your mindfulness back to your breath. Take a couple of additional full breaths, and when you feel prepared, gradually open your eyes.

Benefits:

- Decreases Stress: Helps quiet the brain and diminish uneasiness.

- Advances Relaxation: Upgrades in general mental and close-to-home prosperity.

- Further develops Focus: Helps clear the brain and further develop fixation.

Day 5: Upgrading Supplement Ingestion

Welcome to Day 5 of your 7-day Transformation venture! The present spotlight is on improving supplement retention, an urgent move toward boosting the advantages of the quality food sources you're eating. Supplement ingestion is impacted by different elements, including the kinds of food sources you eat, their blends, and your gut-related well-being. By picking feasts and practices that help ideal assimilation, you'll guarantee your body gets the full range of nutrients, minerals, and other fundamental supplements it necessities to flourish.

Breakfast: Green Smoothie

Begin your day with a supplement thick Green Smoothie. This smoothie is intended to be effectively edible, taking into consideration the most extreme ingestion of nutrients and minerals.

Ingredients:

- 1 cup spinach leaves

- 1 cup kale leaves (stems eliminated)

- 1 banana

- 1/2 cup pineapple pieces

- 1/2 avocado

- 1 tablespoon chia seeds

- 1 tablespoon ground flaxseeds

- 1 cup almond milk or coconut water

- 1 teaspoon spirulina powder (discretionary)

Instructions:

1. Join all fixings in a blender.

2. Mix until smooth and rich.

3. Fill a glass and appreciate right away.

Benefits:

- Spinach and Kale: High in nutrients A, C, K, and folate.

- Banana and Pineapple: Give regular pleasantness and gut-related chemicals.

- Avocado: Adds solid fats, which help in the retention of fat-dissolvable nutrients.

- Chia and Flaxseeds: Wealthy in fiber and omega-3 unsaturated fats.

- Spirulina: Offers extra protein and supplements.

This green smoothie isn't just reviving but is additionally loaded with supplements that are handily retained, setting major areas of strength for an establishment for your day.

Lunch: Lentil Soup

For lunch, partake in a good and feeding Lentil Soup. Lentils are an incredible wellspring of protein, fiber, and fundamental supplements that help processing and supplement ingestion.

Ingredients:

- 1 tablespoon olive oil

- 1 onion, cleaved

- 2 garlic cloves, minced

- 2 carrots, cleaved

- 2 celery stems, cleaved

- 1 cup dried lentils, washed

- 1 can (14.5 oz) diced tomatoes

- 4 cups vegetable stock

- 1 teaspoon cumin

- 1 teaspoon turmeric

- 1 teaspoon paprika

- Salt and pepper to taste

- 1 cup spinach leaves

- Juice of 1 lemon

- New parsley for embellish

Instructions:

1. Heat olive oil in a huge pot over medium intensity. Add onion and garlic, and sauté until fragrant.

2. Add carrots and celery, and cook until delicate.

3. Mix in lentils, diced tomatoes, vegetable stock, cumin, turmeric, paprika, salt, and pepper.

4. Heat to the point of boiling, then lessen intensity and stew for 25-30 minutes, or until lentils are delicate.

5. Add spinach leaves and cook until shriveled.

6. Mix in lemon squeeze and embellish with new parsley before serving.

Benefits:

- Lentils: High in protein, fiber, and iron.

- Vegetables: Give a scope of nutrients and minerals.

- Spices: Cumin and turmeric have mitigating and gut-related benefits.

- Lemon Juice: Improves iron ingestion from lentils.

This lentil soup is both consoling and nutritious, offering an abundance of effectively absorbable supplements.

Supper: Heated Chicken with Broiled Vegetables

End your day with a basic yet tasty Heated Chicken with Cooked Vegetables. This dinner is plentiful in protein, fiber, and different nutrients and minerals that help general well-being and supplement assimilation.

Ingredients:

- 2 boneless, skinless chicken bosoms

- 1 tablespoon olive oil

- 1 teaspoon dried rosemary

- 1 teaspoon dried thyme

- Salt and pepper to taste

- 1 cup child carrots

- 1 cup Brussels sprouts, divided

- 1 cup butternut squash, cubed

- 1 red onion, cleaved

- 2 tablespoons balsamic vinegar

Instructions:

1. Preheat the broiler to 400°F (200°C).

2. Put chicken bosoms on a baking sheet. Sprinkle with olive oil and season with rosemary, thyme, salt, and pepper.

3. Organize child carrots, Brussels sprouts, butternut squash, and red onion around the chicken. Shower with balsamic vinegar.

4. Broil on the stove for 25-30 minutes, or until the chicken is cooked through and the vegetables are delicate.

5. Serve right away, matching each part of the chicken with a liberal aid of broiled vegetables.

Benefits:

- Chicken: Gives fit protein, fundamental for muscle fix and development.

- Vegetables: High in fiber, nutrients, and minerals.

- Olive Oil and Balsamic Vinegar: Add sound fats and improve the assimilation of fat-solvent nutrients.

This feast is adjusted and tasty, guaranteeing you end your day with a supplement stuffed supper.

Work out: Extreme cardio exercise (HIIT)

Consolidate Extreme cardio exercise (HIIT) into your daily schedule to help your digestion and backing generally speaking well-being. HIIT includes short explosions of serious activity followed by times of rest or low-power workouts, advancing cardiovascular well-being, and effective calorie consumption.

Routine:

1. Warm-Up: 5-10 minutes of light cardio, like energetic strolling or running.

2. HIIT Circuit:

   - Bouncing Jacks: 30 seconds on, 30 seconds rest

   - Burpees: 30 seconds on, 30 seconds rest

   - Mountain Climbers: 30 seconds on, 30 seconds rest

- Squat Jumps: 30 seconds on, 30 seconds rest

   - Plank: Hold for 1 moment

3. Cool-Down: 5-10 minutes of extending to loosen up your muscles.

Benefits:

- Helps Metabolism: Increments calorie consumption and works on metabolic rate.

- Upgrades Cardiovascular Health: Further develops heart and lung capability.

- Develops Fortitude and Endurance: Advances by and large wellness.

Care: Appreciation Practice

End your day with a care practice that spotlights the appreciation. Appreciation practice helps shift your concentration to positive parts of your life, lessening pressure and upgrading general prosperity.

Work out: Appreciation Journaling

1. Track down a peaceful, agreeable spot to sit with your diary and a pen.

2. Think about your day and record three things you are thankful for. These can be straightforward minutes, huge accomplishments, or anything that gives you pleasure.

3. Expound on why you are appreciative of everything, zeroing in on the sentiments and encounters related to them.

4. Take a couple of full breaths, permitting yourself to encounter the feeling of appreciation completely.

Benefits:

- Lessens Stress: Assists shift with centering from negative to positive, diminishing tension.

- Advances Happiness: Improves in a general state of mind and prosperity.

- Works on Mental Health: Empowers an uplifting perspective on life.

Day 6: Streamlining Gut Wellbeing

Welcome to Day 6 of your extraordinary excursion! The present spotlight is on improving gut well-being, a basic part of by and large health. A solid gut impacts processing as well as the invulnerable framework, emotional wellness, and even weight of the stomach. By consolidating gut cordial food varieties, participating in proactive tasks, and rehearsing care, you'll uphold your gut-related framework and improve your body's capacity to work at its ideal.

Breakfast: Chia Seed Pudding

Begin your day with a nutritious and heavenly Chia Seed Pudding. This morning meal is loaded with fiber, omega-3 unsaturated fats, and cell reinforcements, which are all useful for gut wellbeing.

Ingredients:

- 3 tablespoons chia seeds

- 1 cup almond milk (or any plant-based milk)

- 1 tablespoon maple syrup or honey

- 1/2 teaspoon vanilla concentrate

- New berries (blueberries, raspberries, strawberries)

- Cut almonds or granola for fixing

Instructions:

1. In a bowl, consolidate chia seeds, almond milk, maple syrup or honey, and vanilla concentrate.

2. Mix well to guarantee chia seeds are uniformly conveyed.

3. Cover and refrigerate for the time being or for no less than 4 hours until the combination thickens into a pudding-like consistency.

4. Before serving, mix the pudding once more top it with new berries, and cut almonds or granola.

Benefits:

- Chia Seeds: High in fiber, which advances sound absorption and ordinary defecations.

- Almond Milk: Gives a smooth base without dairy, which can be gainful for those with lactose prejudice.

- Berries: Plentiful in cell reinforcements and nutrients, adding to in general destroys wellbeing.

This chia seed pudding is simply difficult to get ready yet in addition a gut-accommodating method for beginning your day, giving dependable energy and satiety.

Lunch: Avocado and Bean Salad

For lunch, partake in a dynamic and fulfilling Avocado and Bean Salad. This salad consolidates different gut well-disposed fixings that offer a scope of supplements and back a sound gut-related framework.

Ingredients:

- 1 avocado, diced

- 1 cup dark beans, depleted and flushed

- 1 cup corn bits (new, canned, or frozen)

- 1 red ringer pepper, cleaved

- 1 little red onion, finely cleaved

- 1 cup cherry tomatoes, split

- 1/4 cup new cilantro, hacked

- Juice of 1 lime

- 2 tablespoons olive oil

- Salt and pepper to taste

Instructions:

1. In a huge bowl, combine avocado, dark beans, corn, ringer pepper, red onion, cherry tomatoes, and cilantro.

2. In a little bowl, whisk together lime juice, olive oil, salt, and pepper.

3. Pour the dressing over the serving of mixed greens and throw tenderly to consolidate.

4. Serve right away or refrigerate for as long as 2 hours before serving.

Benefits:

- Avocado: Gives solid fats and fiber, which help in supplement assimilation and gut wellbeing.

- Dark Beans: High in fiber and protein, supporting a sound gut-related framework.

- Corn and Chime Pepper: Offer extra fiber, nutrients, and cell reinforcements.

- Lime Juice and Olive Oil: Improve flavor and backing generally gut-related well-being.

This salad is a bright and nutritious choice for lunch, loaded with fixings that advance a sound gut.

Supper: Shrimp and Veggie Sautéed food

End your day with a delightful and nutritious Shrimp and Veggie Sautéed food. This supper is plentiful in protein, fiber, and various nutrients and minerals, all of which add to a sound gut.

Ingredients:

- 1 pound shrimp, stripped and deveined

- 1 tablespoon coconut oil or olive oil

- 2 garlic cloves, minced

- 1 inch ginger, ground

- 1 red chile pepper, cut

- 1 zucchini, cut

- 1 cup snap peas

- 1 cup broccoli florets

- 2 tablespoons soy sauce or tamari

- 1 tablespoon sesame oil

- 1 tablespoon sesame seeds

- Cooked earthy-colored rice or quinoa for serving

Instructions:

1. Heat coconut oil in a huge skillet or wok over medium-high intensity.

2. Add garlic and ginger, and sauté until fragrant.

3. Add shrimp and cook until pink and misty, around 2-3 minutes. Eliminate shrimp from the skillet and put away.

4. In a similar skillet, add red chime pepper, zucchini, snap peas, and broccoli. Pan sear for 5-7 minutes or until vegetables is delicate and fresh.

5. Return the shrimp to the skillet and add soy sauce or tamari and sesame oil.

6. Sprinkle with sesame seeds before serving.

7. Serve over cooked earthy colored rice or quinoa.

Benefits:

- Shrimp: Gives slender protein, fundamental for muscle fix and general well-being.

- Vegetables: High in fiber, nutrients, and cell reinforcements, supporting gut wellbeing.

- Soy Sauce or Tamari: Adds umami flavor without the gluten (tamari is sans gluten).

- Sesame Oil and Seeds: Offer solid fats and extra supplements.

This sautéed food is a fast, delightful, and supplement thick supper choice that upholds a sound gut and in general well-being.

Work out: Dance Exercise

Integrate a Dance Exercise into your day to help your mindset, and work on cardiovascular well-being, and back gut-related capability. Moving is a tomfoolery and connecting method for remaining dynamic and can be adjusted to any wellness level.

Routine:

1. Warm-Up: 5-10 minutes of delicate extending and light development to set up your body.

2. Dance Session: 30-45 minutes of moving to your number one music. You can follow a dance exercise video or free-form.

3. Cool-Down: 5-10 minutes of extending to loosen up your muscles and lower your pulse.

Benefits:

- Cardiovascular Health: Further develops heart and lung capability.

- Mindset Enhancement: Deliveries endorphins, decreasing pressure and advancing joy.

- Gut-related Support: Active work can help with absorption and forestall stoppage.

A dance exercise is an upbeat method for remaining dynamic and advancing general well-being, including a solid gut-related framework.

Care: Moderate Muscle Unwinding

End your day with a care practice zeroed in on Moderate Muscle Unwinding (PMR). PMR is a procedure that includes straining and afterward loosening up each muscle bunch in your body, advancing unwinding, and diminishing pressure.

Work out: Moderate Muscle Relaxation

1. Track down a calm, agreeable spot to sit or rest.

2. Shut your eyes and take a couple of full breaths, zeroing in on the vibe of the air entering and leaving your body.

3. Begin with your feet. Tense the muscles in your feet by twisting your toes and holding the strain for 5-10 seconds.

4. Discharge the strain and notice the sensation of unwinding in your feet.

5. Climb to your calves. Tense the muscles by arching your foot and holding the strain for 5-10 seconds.

Benefits:

- Diminishes Stress: Helps discharge actual strain and advances a feeling of quiet.

- Further develops Sleep: Advances unwinding, making it more straightforward to nod off.

- Upgrades Body Awareness: Builds attention to where you hold strain in your body.

Day 7: Accomplishing Full-Body Transformation

Welcome to the last day of your groundbreaking process! Day 7 is tied in with accomplishing a full-body Transformation and considering the headway you've made throughout the last week. Today, you will zero in on supplement-rich feasts, a full-body extending routine to improve adaptability and unwinding, and care practices to harden your achievements and plan for what's to come.

Breakfast: Berry and Nut Smoothie

Begin your last day with a Berry and Nut Smoothie, a delectable and supplement-pressed method for filling your body. This smoothie is stacked with cancer prevention agents, solid fats, and protein to launch your day and back your Transformation.

Ingredients:

- 1 cup blended berries (blueberries, strawberries, raspberries)

- 1 banana

- 1/2 cup Greek yogurt or plant-based yogurt

- 1/4 cup crude almonds or pecans

- 1 tablespoon chia seeds

- 1 tablespoon almond spread or peanut butter

- 1 cup almond milk or other plant-based milk

- 1 teaspoon honey or maple syrup (discretionary)

Instructions:

1. Consolidate all fixings in a blender.

2. Mix until smooth and velvety.

3. Fill a glass and appreciate right away.

Benefits:

- Berries: High in cell reinforcements and nutrients, supporting safe well-being and lessening aggravation.

- Greek Yogurt: Gives protein and probiotics,, supporting gut wellbeing and satiety.

- Nuts and Nut Butter: Offer sound fats and extra protein, advancing supported energy and supplement retention.

- Chia Seeds: Wealthy in omega-3 unsaturated fats and fiber, supporting assimilation and by and large wellbeing.

This smoothie is an ideal equilibrium between flavors and supplements, giving a strong beginning to your last day of Transformation.

Lunch: Rainbow Veggie Bowl

For lunch, partake in a lively and sustaining Rainbow Veggie Bowl. This bowl joins various vivid vegetables, each offering one-of-a-kind supplements that help in general well-being and health.

Ingredients:

- 1 cup cooked quinoa or earthy-colored rice

- 1/2 cup red cabbage, destroyed

- 1/2 cup carrots, ground

- 1/2 cup cherry

Tomatoes split

- 1/2 cup cucumber, diced

- 1/2 cup chickpeas, depleted and washed

- 1/2 avocado, cut

- 2 tablespoons sunflower seeds or pumpkin seeds

- New cilantro or parsley for embellish

Dressing:

- 2 tablespoons tahini

- Juice of 1 lemon

- 1 tablespoon apple juice vinegar

- 1 tablespoon olive oil

- 1 teaspoon maple syrup or honey

- Salt and pepper to taste

Instructions:

1. In an enormous bowl, organize the cooked quinoa or earthy-colored rice as the base.

2. Add the red cabbage, carrots, cherry tomatoes, cucumber, chickpeas, and avocado on top.

3. Sprinkle with sunflower seeds or pumpkin seeds and enhance with new cilantro or parsley.

4. In a little bowl, whisk together the dressing fixings until smooth.

5. Shower the dressing over the veggie bowl and throw delicately to join.

Benefits:

- Quinoa/Brown Rice: Give complex carbs and protein, supporting supported energy.

- Vegetables: Offer many nutrients, minerals, and cell reinforcements, advancing generally speaking wellbeing.

- Chickpeas: High in protein and fiber, helping with assimilation and satiety.

- Avocado: Adds solid fats, which support supplement retention and heart well-being.

- Tahini Dressing: Wealthy in sound fats and adds a rich, tasty part to the bowl.

This rainbow veggie bowl is a banquet for the eyes and the body, conveying a range of supplements that add to your general prosperity.

 Supper: Lean Meat with Steamed Vegetables Supper: Lean Meat with Steamed Vegetables

End your day with a basic yet nutritious supper of Lean Meat with Steamed Vegetables. This feast gives top-notch protein and various vegetables that help your body change.

Ingredients:

- 2 lean chicken bosoms, turkey cutlets, or fish filets

- 1 tablespoon olive oil

- 1 teaspoon dried spices (thyme, rosemary, or oregano)

- Salt and pepper to taste

- 1 cup broccoli florets

- 1 cup cauliflower florets

- 1 cup green beans

- 1 tablespoon lemon juice

- New spices for embellish (parsley, dill, or basil)

Instructions:

1. Preheat the stove to 375°F (190°C).

2. Put the rest meat on a baking sheet, shower with olive oil, and season with dried spices, salt, and pepper.

3. Heat in the preheated broiler for 20-25 minutes, or until the meat is cooked through.

4. While the meat is heating up, steam the broccoli, cauliflower, and green beans until delicate.

5. Organize the steamed vegetables on a plate and shower with lemon juice.

6. Serve the heated meat close by the vegetables, decorating with new spices.

Benefits:

- Lean Meat: Gives great protein, fundamental for muscle fix and support.

- Steamed Vegetables: Plentiful in nutrients, minerals, and fiber, supporting the processing and generally speaking wellbeing.

- Olive Oil and Lemon Juice: Add flavor and sound fats, improving supplement assimilation.

This supper is a decent and nutritious method for closing your last day, furnishing your body with the fundamental supplements it necessities to flourish.

Work out: Full-Body Extending

Integrate a Full-Body Extending routine into your day to upgrade adaptability, further develop flow, and advance unwinding. Extending assuages muscle strain and readies your body for proceeding with movement.

Routine:

1. Warm-Up: 5-10 minutes of light cardio, like strolling or running set up.

2. Full-Body Stretching:

  - Neck Stretch: Slant your head aside, bringing your ear toward your shoulder. Hold for 20-30 seconds and rehash on the opposite side.

  - Shoulder Stretch: Arrive at one arm across your body and utilize the contrary hand to pull it nearer to your chest tenderly. Hold for 20-30 seconds and rehash on the opposite side.

  - Chest Stretch: Fasten your hands behind your back and lift your arms somewhat, opening your chest. Hold for 20-30 seconds.

  - Upper Back Stretch: Broaden your arms before you, catching your hands together. Round your back and push your hands forward, extending the upper back. Hold for 20-30 seconds.

- Side Stretch: Stand with your feet shoulder-width separated. Arrive at one arm above and shelter the opposite side, extending the side of your body. Hold for 20-30 seconds and rehash on the opposite side.

- Hamstring Stretch: Sit on the floor with one leg broadened and the other twisted. Reach toward your toes on the lengthy leg, extending the hamstring. Hold for 20-30 seconds and rehash on the opposite side.

- Quad Stretch: Stand on one leg, pulling the contrary foot toward your rump to extend the quadriceps. Hold for 20-30 seconds and rehash on the opposite side.

Benefits:

- Further develops Flexibility: Improves the scope of movement in your joints.

- Advances Circulation: Increments blood stream to muscles and tissues.

- Alleviates Muscle Tension: Lessens firmness and distress in muscles.

Full-body extending is a delicate and successful method for finishing up your active work, advancing unwinding, and setting up your body for tranquil rest.

Care: Reflection and Preparing

End your day and your 7-day change venture with a care practice zeroed in all things considered and preparing. This training assists you with recognizing your accomplishments, distinguishing regions for development, and putting forth objectives for what's to come.

Work out: Reflection and Planning

1. Track down a tranquil, agreeable spot to sit or rest.

2. Shut your eyes and take a couple of full breaths, focusing on yourself right now.

3. Consider the previous week. Think about the accompanying inquiries:

   - What were your most critical achievements?

   - What difficulties did you face, and how could you conquer them?

   - How would you feel actually, intellectually, and sincerely contrasted with the start of the week?

4. Record your appearance in a diary, zeroing in on both positive encounters and examples learned.

5. Recognize regions where you can keep on moving along. Put forth practical and explicit objectives for the next few long p.

Benefits:

- **Upgrades Self-Awareness:** Supports reflection on self-improvement and accomplishments.

- **Advances Objective Setting:** Recognizes future targets and arranges progress.

- **Decreases Stress:** Encourages a feeling of quiet and reason.

CHAPTER 5: Supporting Your Transformation

Congrats on finishing your 7-day change venture! As you push ahead, supporting the advancement you've accomplished is essential. Part 5 spotlights on long-haul feast arranging systems to assist you with keeping a sound way of life and receiving the rewards of your change.

5.11 Long-haul Feast Arranging

Long-haul feast arranging is the foundation of supporting your change. By making an organized way to deal with sustenance, you can guarantee that smart dieting turns into a feasible propensity as opposed to an impermanent exertion. Here are key methodologies to assist you with arranging your feasts really:

1. Laying out Good dieting Examples

Building an underpinning of smart dieting designs is fundamental for long-haul achievement. Consider integrating the accompanying standards into your feast arranging:

Adjusted Meals: Incorporate various food varieties from all nutrition classes — organic products, vegetables, entire grains, lean proteins, and sound fats — to guarantee you're getting a great many supplements.

- **Segment Control:** Be aware of piece sizes to keep a solid weight and forestall gorging.

- Customary Meals: Go for the gold dinners each day with solid snacks depending on the situation to keep up with energy levels and forestall desires.

- Hydration: Drink a lot of water over the day to help with processing, hydration, and in general well-being.

2. Week by week Feast Prep

Feast preparing saves time and guarantees that sound choices are promptly accessible, diminishing the compulsion to select less nutritious decisions when you're occupied or tired. This is the way to integrate feast prep into your daily schedule:

- Pick a Day: Devote one day out of each week to design and set up your feasts. This could include shopping for food, bunch cooking proteins and grains, and hacking vegetables.

- Storage: Put resources into quality food stockpiling holders to store prepared dinners and tidbits. Partition feasts into individual bits for simple in and out choices.

- Variety: Set up various dinners and snacks to keep your feasts fascinating consistently. Utilize different cooking techniques and flavors to add flavor without overabundance of calories.

3. Accentuating Supplement Thick Food sources

Center around supplement thick food varieties that give fundamental nutrients, minerals, and cancer prevention agents while supporting general well-being and prosperity:

- Vegetables: Mean to fill half of your plate with bright vegetables at every dinner. They're low in calories and high in fiber, advancing satiety and stomach-related well-being.

- Lean Proteins: Integrate lean protein sources like poultry, fish, tofu, beans, and vegetables. Protein upholds muscle fix, safe capability, and generally cell wellbeing.

- Entire Grains: Pick entire grains like quinoa, earthy colored rice, oats, and entire wheat bread over refined grains. They give fiber and fundamental supplements to support energy.

4. Adaptability and Versatility

Keeping a sound eating regimen doesn't mean wiping out all guilty pleasures or severe adherence to an inflexible feast plan. Permit yourself adaptability and flexibility:

- Periodic Treats: Consolidate incidental treats or most loved food varieties with some restraint to stay away from sensations of hardship.

- Adjustments: Be adaptable with your dinner plan in light of changes in timetable, inclinations, or exceptional events. Adjust recipes and dinner thoughts to suit your requirements while remaining within your nourishing objectives.

5. Looking for Help and Responsibility

Draw in with an emotionally supportive network or responsibility accomplice to remain propelled and focused on your drawn-out objectives:

- Family and Friends: Offer dinners and solid recipes with loved ones who support your excursion to keep up with inspiration and motivation.

- Online Communities: Join online discussions, virtual entertainment gatherings, or applications zeroed in on smart dieting and dinner-making arrangements for extra help and support.

5.12 Integrating Activity into Your Everyday Daily practice

Practice is an essential part of keeping up with your change and in general prosperity. By integrating actual work into your everyday daily practice, you can upgrade your well-being, work on your state of mind, and support the advancement you've accomplished. In this section, we'll investigate useful techniques for coordinating activity flawlessly into your life for long-haul achievement.

Figuring out the Significance of Activity

Standard activity offers a bunch of advantages for both physical and emotional well-being. Here are a few justifications for why integrating exercise into your day-to-day schedule is fundamental:

- Weight Management: Exercise assists consume calories, working with muscles, and keep a sound weight, decreasing the gamble of stoutness-related medical issues.

- Cardiovascular Health: Actual work fortifies the heart and further develops course, bringing down the gamble of coronary illness, stroke, and hypertension.

- Muscle Strength and Bone Health: Obstruction preparing practices assemble bulk and increment bone thickness, decreasing the gamble of osteoporosis and breaks.

- Mental Well-being: Exercise discharges endorphins, synapses that advance sensations of bliss and decrease pressure, uneasiness, and despondency.

- Further developed Sleep: Standard active work can further develop rest quality and span, prompting better general rest and recuperation.

Procedures for Integrating Activity

Integrating exercise into your day-to-day schedule doesn't need to be overwhelming or tedious. With the right methodology and mentality, you can track down pleasant ways of moving your body and receive the rewards of actual work. Here are a few pragmatic procedures to assist you with beginning:

1. Find Exercises You Appreciate

The way to stay with a workout routine is to track down exercises that you appreciate. Whether it's moving, climbing, swimming, or yoga, pick exercises that cause you to feel better and keep you spurred to move. Try different things with various sorts of activity until you find what impacts you.

2. Make It Helpful

Eliminate obstructions to practice by making it as helpful as could be expected. Pick exercises that fit flawlessly into your everyday daily practice, whether it's going for a stroll during your mid-day break, cycling to work, or doing a speedy exercise at home. The simpler it is to integrate practice into your life, the more certain you are to stay with it.

3. Put forth Sensible Objectives

Put forth practical and attainable objectives that line up with your wellness level and way of life. Whether it's strolling 10,000 stages per day, running a 5K, or dominating another yoga present, laying out unambiguous objectives gives you something to pursue and helps keep tabs on your development after some time.

4. Plan It

Deal with practice like some other significant arrangement and timetable it into your schedule. Shut out time for actual work every day, whether it's in the first part of the day, evening, or night. By focusing on exercise and making it a non-debatable piece of your day, you're bound to see everything through to completion.

5. Stir It Up

Keep your workout routine new and energizing by stirring up your exercises consistently. Consolidate various exercises, for example, cardio, strength preparation, adaptability, and equilibrium workout, to work different muscle gatherings and forestall fatigue. Attempt new classes, outside exercises, or exercise recordings to keep things intriguing.

6. Make It Social

Practice with companions, relatives, or colleagues to make it more agreeable and social. Join a games group, wellness class, or climbing gathering to interface with other people who share your inclinations and give inspiration and responsibility.

7. Be Adaptable

Life can be erratic, and there will be days when your exercise plans go off track. Be adaptable and ready to adjust to changes in your timetable or conditions. On the off chance that you miss an exercise, don't harp on it — simply take up where you left out and continue to push ahead.

8. Pay attention to Your Body

Focus on your body's signs and change your workout routine in like manner. If you're feeling exhausted or encountering torment or distress, take a rest day or pick a lower-force movement. Pushing through agony can prompt injury and misfortunes, so focus on well-being and taking care of oneself.

5.13 Care Practices for Lasting Change

Care is a strong practice that can improve your capacity to support the positive changes you've made during your change process. By developing present-second mindfulness and non-critical acknowledgment, care assists you with remaining associated with your objectives, overseeing pressure, and pursuing cognizant decisions that help your prosperity. In this part, we'll investigate different care rehearses that you can coordinate into your routine to cultivate enduring change.

Figuring out Care

Care is the act of being completely present and taking part in the occasion, without judgment or interruption. It includes focusing on your viewpoints, feelings, and sensations as they emerge, noticing them without appending to them or responding imprudently. Research has demonstrated the way that customary care practice can decrease pressure, work on close-to-home guidelines, improve concentration and consideration, and advance generally speaking prosperity.

Advantages of Care for Supporting Your Change

With regards to supporting your change, care offers a few key advantages that help long-haul achievement:

Stress Reduction: Care lessens the physiological and mental impacts of pressure, advancing a feeling of quiet and unwinding.

- Profound Regulation: By developing consciousness of your feelings, care empowers you to answer difficulties and mishaps with more prominent flexibility and lucidity.

- Upgraded Self-Awareness: Care increments mindfulness, assisting you with perceiving examples of conduct, considerations, and feelings that might influence your well-being and prosperity.

- Further developed Choice Making: By encouraging present-second mindfulness, care upgrades your capacity to settle on cognizant decisions lined up with your objectives and values.

- Expanded Satisfaction: Care supports appreciation and appreciation for the current second, cultivating a feeling of satisfaction and fulfillment in your day-to-day existence.

Pragmatic Care Practices

Coordinating care into your everyday schedule doesn't need long stretches of reflection or specific preparation. Basic, open practices can significantly affect your prosperity and capacity to support positive changes. The following are a few care practices to investigate:

1. Careful Relaxing

Careful breathing is a primary practice that helps anchor your mindfulness right now and quiet the brain. This is the way to rehearse careful relaxing:

- Find an agreeable position: Sit or rest in an agreeable position, with your back straight yet not unbending.
- Close your eyes: Shut your eyes or relax your look.
- Zero in on your breath: Carry your consideration regarding the vibe of your breath as it enters and leaves your nose or fills your lungs.
- Notice without judgment: Notice any considerations, feelings, or impressions that emerge, permitting them to

travel every which way without becoming involved with them.

- Remain present: Assuming that your brain meanders, tenderly take your concentration back to your breath. Go on for a few minutes, continuously broadening the length as you become more OK with the training.

Careful breathing can be drilled anyplace, whenever, and fills in as an establishing procedure during snapshots of stress or overpowering.

2. Body Output Reflection

Body filter reflection includes deliberately paying attention to various pieces of your body, and seeing sensations without judgment. This is the way to rehearse a body examination:

- ✓ Rests or sits comfortably: Find a peaceful space where you can unwind without interruptions.
- ✓ Begin at your feet: Carry your thoughtfulness regarding your toes, seeing any sensations like warmth, shivering, or strain.
- ✓ Progress slowly: Move your consideration step by step up through your feet, legs, middle, arms, and head, seeing sensations in every space.
- ✓ Discharge tension: Assuming you notice strain or distress, inhale into that area and intentionally loosen up it.
- ✓ Entire body awareness: Whenever you've examined your whole body, carry your attention to your body in general, seeing how it feels at this time.

Body examination contemplation can assist with delivering actual strain, further develop body mindfulness, and advance unwinding.

3. Careful Eating

Careful eating includes focusing on full the experience of eating, from picking your food to enjoying each nibble. This pursuit energizes better eating routines and food satisfaction. This is the way to rehearse careful eating:

- Draw in your senses: Notice the tones, surfaces, and scents of your food before taking a nibble.
- Eat slowly: Take little chomps and bite completely, focusing on the flavors and surfaces in your mouth.
- Stop between bites: Put down your utensils among nibbles and check in with your yearning and completion signals.
- Be present: Limit interruptions like screens or perusing materials while eating, zeroing in exclusively on the demonstration of eating.
- Express gratitude: Pause for a minute to see the value in the sustenance your food gives and develop appreciation for the dinner.

Careful eating cultivates a better relationship with food, upgrades processing, and advances careful food decisions.

4. Strolling Contemplation

Strolling contemplation consolidates care with actual development, permitting you to develop mindfulness while strolling. This training should be possible inside or outside at an agreeable speed. This is the way to work on strolling reflection:

- Pick a location: Find a peaceful spot where you can walk continuously, like a recreation area or calm neighborhood road.

- ❖ Set an intention: Start with a couple of moments of careful breathing to focus yourself and set an aim for your walk.
- ❖ Walk mindfully: Begin strolling at a sluggish, conscious speed, focusing on the impression of your feet contacting the ground.
- ❖ Notice surroundings: Notice the sights, sounds, and scents around you without judgment or connection.
- ❖ Get back to the present: Assuming that your brain meanders, delicately take your concentration back to the vibe of strolling and your environmental elements.
- ❖ End mindfully: Steadily sluggish your speed as you approach the finish of your walk, taking a couple of seconds to consider your experience before closing.

Strolling contemplation advances active work, stress decreases, and association with the normal world.

5. Appreciation Practice

Rehearsing appreciation includes purposefully zeroing in on the positive parts of your life and communicating appreciation for them. This training develops a positive mentality and upgrades in general prosperity. This is the way to rehearse appreciation:

- ➤ Everyday reflection: Take a couple of seconds every day to consider three things you're thankful for. These can be straightforward joys, snapshots of association, or individual accomplishments.
- ➤ Appreciation journal: Keep an appreciation diary where you record things you're thankful for every day or week. Consider the reason why these things are significant to you.
- ➤ Offer appreciation: Express thanks to others by saying thanks to them for their generosity, backing, or commitment to your life. This should be possible

verbally, through a manually written note, or using text/email.

Appreciation practice improves inspiration, flexibility, and close-to-home prosperity, supporting your excursion towards supported change.

6. Careful Correspondence

Careful correspondence includes listening effectively, talking deliberately, and answering nicely in discussions. This training cultivates further associations, lessens misconceptions, and advances sympathy and understanding. This is the way to rehearse careful correspondence:

- Listen fully: Offer the speaker your full consideration, keeping in touch and staying away from interruptions.
- Stop before responding: Pause for a minute to consider your contemplations and sentiments before answering. This assists you with conveying all the more plainly and truly.
- Practice empathy: Come at the situation from the other individual's perspective, looking to figure out their point of view and sentiments without judgment.
- Talk mindfully: Express yourself deliberately, taking into account their effect on the audience. Use "I" proclamations to offer your viewpoints and sentiments.

Careful correspondence upgrades connections, advances compelling compromise, and encourages a strong climate for self-improvement.

CHAPTER 6: Investigating and Changes

Congrats on leaving on your groundbreaking process! As you explore the way toward a better, more slender you, it's fundamental to recognize that difficulties might emerge en route. In Part 6, we'll investigate normal hindrances you could experience and give commonsense answers to assist you with defeating them, guaranteeing that you keep focused on your objectives.

6.11 Common challenges and solutions

1. Absence of Inspiration

Challenge: It's normal to encounter variances in inspiration, particularly when confronted with obstructions or misfortunes.

Solution:

a. Return to Your Why: Help yourself to remember the motivations behind why you began this excursion in any case. Whether it's working on your well-being, helping your certainty, or setting a positive model for friends and family, reconnecting with your fundamental inspirations can reignite your drive.

b. Set Little, Attainable Goals: Separate your bigger objectives into more modest, more sensible achievements. Praise every accomplishment en route to keep up with force and keep inspiration levels high.

c. Track down Accountability: Offer your objectives with a companion, relative, or online local area. Having somebody to consider you responsible can offer help and consolation when inspiration fades.

2. Levels

Challenge: After introductory advancement, you might arrive at a level where your weight reduction or wellness objectives slow down.

Solution:

> ➤ Reevaluate Your Habits: Investigate your eating regimen, workout daily practice, and way of life propensities. Are there regions where you can make enhancements or changes?
> ➤ Change Up Your Workouts: Integrate assortment into your workout daily practice by attempting new exercises, expanding power, or zeroing in on various muscle gatherings. This can assist with forestalling fatigue and animate further advancement.
> ➤ Change Your Caloric Intake: As your body changes, your caloric requirements may likewise vary. Consider talking with a nutritionist or dietitian to reconsider your calorie consumption and guarantee it lines up with your objectives.

3. Time Imperatives

Challenge: Adjusting work, family, and different obligations can make it trying to set aside opportunities for exercise and feast planning.

Solution:

- Focus on Self-Care: Perceive the significance of focusing on your well-being and prosperity. Plan committed time for exercise and feast prep, regarding it as non-debatable meetings with yourself.
- Enhance Your Schedule: Search for pockets of time over the day where you can fit in fast exercises or dinner prep

meetings. This could incorporate early mornings, mid-day breaks, or nights after work.

- Consolidate Activities: Performing various tasks can be a helpful technique for squeezing exercise into a bustling timetable. Think about strolling or cycling to work, doing bodyweight practices while staring at the television, or feast preparing while at the same time paying attention to a webcast.

4. Profound Eating

Challenge: Stress, weariness, and different feelings can set off desires and lead to undesirable dietary patterns.

Solution:

- ✓ Practice Careful Eating: Focus on your body's craving and completion signs, eating gradually and relishing each chomp. Careful eating can assist you with turning out to be more mindful of your food decisions and decrease the probability of close-to-home eating.
- ✓ Track down Elective Adapting Mechanisms: Recognize elective ways of adapting to pressure or fatigue that don't include food. This could incorporate activity, reflection, side interests, or investing energy with friends and family.
- ✓ Look for Support: On the off chance that close-to-home eating turns into a repetitive issue, consider looking for help from a specialist or instructor who can assist you with tending to basic profound triggers and foster better survival techniques.

5. Prevailing burden

Challenge: Parties, festivities, and companion impact can make it hard to adhere to your sound propensities.

Solution:

- Impart Your Goals: Open up to loved ones about your well-being and wellness objectives. Tell them how they can uphold you, whether it's by offering better food choices at social occasions or empowering actual work.
- Plan Ahead: Before going to get-togethers, have an arrangement set up for how you'll explore food decisions and oversee enticements. Think about eating a good dinner in advance, carrying a nutritious dish to share, or defining limits around liquor utilization.
- Zero in on Balance: Permit yourself to appreciate periodic extravagances without culpability. Recollect that equilibrium and balance are vital to long-haul achievement, and one feast or occasion will not crash your advancement.

6.12 Changing the Arrangement for Explicit Requirements

1. Ailments

Challenge: People with ailments like diabetes, coronary illness, or food sensitivities might require exceptional contemplation while following a well-being and health plan.

Solution:

- Talk with a Medical Services Professional: Before rolling out any huge improvements to your eating regimen or workout daily schedule, talk with a medical care supplier or enlisted dietitian. They can give customized directions custom-made to your particular requirements and clinical history.
- Change Wholesome Recommendations: Relying upon your ailment, you might have to alter specific parts of your eating regimen, like starch consumption for diabetes the executives or sodium admission for heart wellbeing. Work with a medical care professional to foster a sustenance plan that upholds your general well-being and health objectives.
- Integrate Safe Activity Practices: Assuming you have an ailment that influences your capacity to work out, like joint inflammation or constant agony, look for direction from an actual specialist or exercise physiologist. They can prescribe protected and successful activity adjustments to oblige your necessities and capacities.

2. Dietary Inclinations

Challenge: People following explicit dietary inclinations or ways of life, like vegetarianism, veganism, or sans gluten eat less, may have to make acclimations to the dinner intended to guarantee it lines up with their dietary requirements.

Solution:

- ❖ Change Feast Options: Trade out fixings or make replacements to oblige dietary inclinations or limitations. For instance, supplant creature proteins with plant-based other options, use sans gluten grains and flours, or consolidate without dairy choices for people with lactose bigotry.
- ❖ Investigate Recipe Modifications: Examination with altering recipes to suit your dietary inclinations while as yet keeping up with nourishing equilibrium. Get innovative with flavor blends and fixing replacements to keep dinners energizing and fulfilling.
- ❖ Look for Recipe Inspiration: Search for recipe motivation from cookbooks, online assets, or web-based entertainment stages custom-fitted to your dietary inclinations. There is an abundance of assets accessible for people following veggie lovers, vegetarians, without gluten, and other particular weight control plans.

3. Spending plan Requirements

Challenge: Following well-being and health anticipate a strict spending plan can introduce difficulties with regards to buying nutritious food sources and getting to wellness assets.

Solution:

- ➢ Plan Dinners Strategically: Make a week-after-week feast plan given spending plan cordial fixings like beans, lentils, entire grains, and occasional produce. Search for deals, limits, and coupons to augment reserve funds on food.

➢ Embrace Plant-Based Proteins: Consolidate plant-based protein sources like beans, lentils, tofu, and temper into your feasts. These choices are much of the time more reasonable than creature proteins and can give more than adequate nourishment at a lower cost.

➢ Investigate Free Wellness Resources: Exploit free or minimal expense wellness assets, for example, online exercise recordings, outside exercises like strolling or running, or local area wellness classes presented at nearby stops or public venues.

4. Time Imperatives

Challenge: Occupied timetables and time imperatives can make it hard to focus on dinner arrangements and exercise.

Solution:

✓ Cluster Cooking: Devote one day out of each week to group preparing and getting ready feasts ahead of time. This can assist with smoothing out supper time during the week and guarantee you have nutritious choices promptly accessible.

✓ Short Workouts: Consolidate short, extreme focus exercises or span instructional courses that can be finished in 20-30 minutes. These exercises are productive and can be effectively fit into occupied plans.

✓ Multitasking: Search for chances to consolidate practice with different exercises, like strolling or trekking to work, doing bodyweight practices while sitting in front of the television, or enjoying dynamic reprieves during the working day.

5. Age-Related Contemplations

Challenge: As people age, their dietary requirements and actual abilities might change, expecting acclimations to their well-being and health plan.

Solution:

- Center around Supplement Density: Choose supplement thick food varieties that give fundamental nutrients, minerals, and cell reinforcements to help generally speaking well-being and prosperity. Consolidate different vivid products of the soil, lean proteins, entire grains, and sound fats into your eating routine.
- Adjust Exercise Routines: Alter workout schedules to oblige age-related changes in portability, adaptability, and strength. Center around low-influence exercises like strolling, swimming, yoga, or jujitsu that are delicate on the joints and advance adaptability and equilibrium.
- Focus on Safety: Focus on security contemplations while working out, for example, utilizing legitimate structure, staying away from high-influence developments that might expand the gamble of injury, and paying attention to your body's signals to keep away from overexertion.

6. Psychological wellness Contemplations

Challenge: People battling with emotional well-being issues like sorrow, uneasiness, or stress might find it trying to keep a well-being and health plan.

Solution:

- Consolidate Care Practices: Coordinate care practices like reflection, profound breathing activities, or yoga into your day-to-day schedule to advance unwinding and lessen pressure.

- Search Support: Contact an emotional wellness expert or instructor for help and direction if you're battling with psychological well-being issues. They can give survival methods, restorative intercessions, and assets to assist you with overseeing side effects and keeping up with general prosperity.
- Center around Self-Care: Focus on taking care of oneself through exercises that feed your brain, body, and soul. Participate in exercises that give you pleasure, like investing energy outside, seeking leisure activities, or associating with friends and family.

6.13 Managing Difficulties

1. Perceiving Difficulties

Challenge: Mishaps can appear in different structures, remembering levels for progress, slips in adherence to your arrangement, or surprising impediments that ruin your excursion.

Solution:

- Recognize Your Feelings: It's not unexpected to feel baffled, disheartened, or deterred when confronted with mishaps. Permit yourself to recognize and handle these feelings without judgment.
- Think about the Cause: Carve out the opportunity to consider the variables that added to the difficulty. Was it a pass in inspiration, outer conditions unchangeable as

far as you might be concerned, or ridiculous assumptions? Understanding the underlying driver can assist you with creating systems to address and conquer future mishaps.

2. Developing Versatility

Challenge: Difficulties can test your versatility and capacity to quickly return from affliction.

Solution:

a. Shift Your Perspective: As opposed to reviewing difficulties as disappointments, rethink them as any open doors for development and learning. Embrace the difficulties as significant examples that add to your self-improvement and strength.

b.   Practice Self-Compassion: Be thoughtful to yourself during seasons of misfortune. Offer yourself a similar empathy and understanding you would reach out to a companion confronting comparable difficulties. Recollect that mishaps are a typical piece of the excursion, and they don't characterize your value or potential for progress.

3. Rethinking Objectives

Challenge: Misfortunes might require a reexamination of your objectives and assumptions.

Solution:

i. Set Sensible Expectations: Evaluate whether your objectives are achievable given your ongoing conditions, assets, and timetable. Change your objectives depending on the situation to guarantee they are practical and feasible.

ii. Center around Cycle Goals: Shift your concentration from result-arranged objectives to deal with situated objectives. Rather than focusing on unambiguous results, focus on the everyday propensities and ways of behaving that add to your general achievement.

4. Building an Emotionally supportive network

Challenge: Mishaps can feel disconnected and overpowering without an emotionally supportive network set up.

Solution:

- Search Support: Connect with companions, relatives, or a believed encouraging group of people for consolation, direction, and responsibility. Offering your difficulties to others can give important viewpoints and daily reassurance during troublesome times.
- Join a Community: Consider joining a care group, online gathering, or web-based entertainment local area zeroed in on wellbeing and health. Interfacing with other people who are on a comparable excursion can cultivate a feeling of fellowship and shared help.

5. Critical thinking Procedures

Challenge: Difficulties require proactive critical thinking procedures to recognize arrangements and beat hindrances.

Solution:

- ➢ Recognize Solutions: Separate the misfortune into sensible parts and conceptualize possible arrangements. Think about looking for input from others or talking with specialists to investigate elective methodologies.

> ➢ Foster an Arrangement of Action: Whenever you've recognized likely arrangements, make a game plan illustrating explicit advances you will take to address the difficulty. Set reasonable timetables and benchmarks to keep tabs on your development.
> ➢ Screen Progress: Routinely assess your advancement and change your arrangement depending on the situation given criticism and results. Celebrate little triumphs en route and stay versatile in your way to deal with beating difficulties.

CHAPTER 7: Examples of overcoming adversity

7.11 Genuine Changes

1. Sarah's Excursion to Wellbeing and Imperativeness

Sarah, a 35-year-old showcasing chief and mother of two had battled with weight gain and low energy for a long time. Disappointed by prevailing fashion counts calories that guaranteed handy solutions but neglected to convey enduring outcomes, she chose to adopt an alternate strategy. With direction from a nutritionist, Sarah took on a fair eating plan and zeroed in on entire food varieties, lean proteins, and a lot of vegetables. She integrated ordinary activity into her everyday practice, beginning with Day-to-day strolls and slowly expanding her wellness level.

Throughout a while, Sarah experienced critical upgrades in her energy levels, state of mind, and general prosperity. She shed pounds consistently and saw positive changes in her body organization. By focusing on taking care of oneself and making maintainable way of life changes, Sarah accomplished her weight reduction objectives as well as acquired certainty and reestablished essentialness.

2. James' Change through Careful Eating

James, a 42-year-old IT proficient, battled with profound eating and stress-related weight gain. He frequently went to nourishment for solace during seasons of pressure, which prompted unfortunate dietary patterns and fluctuating weight. Still up in the air to break liberated from this cycle, James signed up for a care-based eating program that trained him to develop mindfulness and presence during dinners.

Through careful eating practices like focusing on yearning and totality signs, enjoying each nibble, and rehearsing appreciation for feeding food sources, James fostered a better relationship with food. He figured out how to oversee pressure all the more successfully through care contemplation and unwinding procedures, which added to better general well-being and prosperity.

James' process featured the significant effect of care on profound dietary patterns and highlighted the significance of addressing basic close-to-home triggers to accomplish enduring change.

7.12 Tributes from Members

1. Emma's Viewpoint on Self-awareness

"Leaving on this groundbreaking excursion has been one of the most remunerating encounters of my life. I've generally battled with fearlessness and self-perception issues, yet through reliable activity, nutritious eating, and a strong local area, I've acquired a newly discovered feeling of strengthening and self-esteem Every little accomplishment en route has built up my confidence in my capacity to make positive change in my life."

2. David's Excursion to Physical and Mental Wellbeing

"Following quite a while of dismissing my well-being, I at long last chose to focus on my prosperity. With direction from a wellness mentor and nutritionist, I fostered a customized plan that lined up with my objectives and way of life. Through normal exercises, adjusted sustenance and care rehearses, I've shed pounds, acquired muscle, and worked on my psychological clearness. This excursion has shown me the significance of taking care of oneself and motivated me to keep a solid way of life as long as possible."

7.13 Master Experiences

1. Nutritionist's Viewpoint on Feasible Dietary Patterns

"Effective change starts with laying out feasible dietary patterns that help long haul wellbeing and prosperity. Centers on eating various supplements and thick food varieties like organic products, vegetables, entire grains, lean proteins, and solid fats. Consolidate careful eating practices to improve consciousness of craving and completion signs, advance processing, and forestall indulging. By focusing on adjusted sustenance and making steady, reasonable changes, people can accomplish enduring outcomes and keep up with their ideal weight."

2. Wellness Coach's Way to Deal with Exercise and Inspiration

"Actual work is fundamental for accomplishing and keeping up with ideal well-being and wellness. Planning a customized practice plan that incorporates a mix of cardiovascular, strength preparation, and adaptability activities can assist people with accomplishing their wellness objectives. Integrate exercises that you appreciate and can support over the long run. Consistency is critical to progress, so find exercises that inspire you and fit into your way of life. Recollect that progress requires some investment, and praise every achievement en route."

Appendix

Recipes for Lively Wellbeing

Smart dieting is the foundation of your excursion to ideal prosperity. In this part, you'll find an assortment of delightful and nutritious recipes intended to feed your body, fulfill your taste buds, and support your well-being objectives. From empowering morning meals to fulfilling suppers and healthy tidbits, these recipes are made with healthy fixings to fuel your change from the back to the front.

Breakfast Recipes

1. Green Smoothie Bowl

   - Fixings:

   - 1 cup spinach

   - 1/2 avocado

   - 1/2 cup frozen berries

   - 1 banana

   - 1 tbsp chia seeds

   - 1 cup almond milk

   - Directions: Mix all fixings until smooth. Top with cut natural products, nuts, and seeds.

2. Chia Seed Pudding

   - Fixings:

   - 1/4 cup chia seeds

- 1 cup almond milk

- 1 tbsp maple syrup

- 1/2 tsp vanilla concentrate

- New berries for garnish

- Guidelines: Blend chia seeds, almond milk, maple syrup, and vanilla concentrate in a bowl. Allow it to sit for 30 minutes or short-term in the fridge. Top with new berries before serving.

Lunch Recipes

1. Quinoa Salad with Lemon-Tahini Dressing

- Fixings:

- 1 cup cooked quinoa

- 1/2 cup chickpeas, depleted and flushed

- 1 cucumber, diced

- 1/2 cup cherry tomatoes, divided

- 1/4 cup slashed new parsley

- Dressing: 2 tbsp tahini, juice of 1 lemon, 1 tbsp olive oil, salt and pepper to taste

Directions: In an enormous bowl, join quinoa, chickpeas, cucumber, tomatoes, and parsley. In a little bowl, whisk together dressing fixings, Pour over salad and prepare to join.

2. Sweet Potato and Dark Bean Tacos

- Fixings:

- 2 enormous yams, diced

- 1 can dark beans, depleted and flushed

- 1 avocado, cut

- Entire grain tortillas

- Discretionary garnishes: salsa, cilantro, lime wedges

- Guidelines: Cook yams on the stove until delicate. Heat dark beans in a skillet until warmed through. Gather tacos with yams, dark beans, avocado cuts, and wanted garnishes.

Supper Recipes

1. Grilled Salmon with Quinoa and Steamed Broccoli

- Fixings:

  - 4 salmon filets

  - 1 cup quinoa, cooked

  - 2 cups broccoli florets

  - Lemon wedges for serving

- Directions: Barbecue salmon filets until cooked through. Present with quinoa and steamed broccoli. Press lemon juice over the salmon before serving.

2. Vegetable Pan fried food with Tofu

- Fixings:

  - 1 block tofu, squeezed and cubed

- Grouped vegetables (chime peppers, broccoli, carrots, snap peas)

  - 2 tbsp soy sauce

- 1 tbsp sesame oil

- 2 cloves garlic, minced

- Cooked earthy colored rice for serving.

- Guidelines: Intensity sesame oil in an enormous skillet or wok. Add tofu and cook until brilliant brown. Add vegetables and garlic, pan sear until delicate. Mix in soy sauce. Serve over earthy colored rice.

Nibble Recipes

1. Homemade Trail Mix

- Fixings:

    - 1 cup blended nuts (almonds, cashews, pecans)

    - 1/2 cup dried organic product (raisins, cranberries)

    - 1/4 cup dim chocolate chips

- Guidelines: Combine all fixings as one in a bowl. Segment into nibble estimated sacks for simple in and out choices.

2. Greek Yogurt with Berries and Honey

- Fixings:

    - 1 cup Greek yogurt

    - Blended berries (strawberries, blueberries, raspberries)

    - Sprinkle of honey

- Guidelines: Spoon Greek yogurt into a bowl. Top with blended berries and sprinkle in with honey.

These recipes are intended to move and support your excursion towards a better way of life. Go ahead and try different things with fixings and adjust recipes to suit your inclinations and dietary requirements.

Shopping Records for Progress

Preparing is vital to keeping a fair and nutritious eating routine. Utilize the accompanying shopping records to stock your kitchen with fundamental elements for planning dinners consistently. Each rundown is coordinated by food class to smooth out your shopping experience and guarantee you have all that you want to follow your feast plan.

Week after week Basic food item Rundown Model

- Produce:

  - Spinach

  - Avocado

  - Berries (strawberries, blueberries, raspberries)

  - Cucumber

  - Cherry tomatoes

  - New parsley

  - Yams

  - Broccoli florets

  - Ringer peppers

  - Carrots

  - Snap peas

- Grains and Legumes:

  - Quinoa

  - Earthy colored rice

  - Entire grain tortillas

- Proteins:

  - Salmon filets

  - Tofu

  - Chickpeas

  - Dark beans

  - Blended nuts (almonds, cashews, pecans)

- Dairy and Alternatives:

  - Greek yogurt

  - Almond milk

- Storeroom Staples:

  - Chia seeds

  - Olive oil

  - Tahini

  - Soy sauce

  - Maple syrup

  - Dim chocolate chips

- Miscellaneous:

- Lemons

- Garlic

- Salsa

- Cilantro

- Honey

Change amounts given your particular feast plan and dietary inclinations. Consolidate occasional produce and investigate neighborhood ranchers' business sectors for new, natural choices whenever the situation allows.

Extra Assets for Proceeded with Help

Changing your way of life is an excursion that requires progressing schooling, motivation, and backing. Investigate the accompanying extra assets to upgrade your insight, find new systems, and interface with a local area of similar people focused on well-being and health.

1. Wellbeing and Health Sites

> ➢ Public Foundations of Wellbeing (NIH): Access dependable data on sustenance, exercise, and wellbeing from a main expert in the biomedical examination.
> ➢ Mayo Clinic: Investigate wellbeing subjects, track down sound recipes, and access health tips from medical care specialists.
> ➢ Harvard Wellbeing Publishing: Find proof-based articles, smart dieting guides, and wellness exhortations from Harvard Clinical School.

2. Wellness Applications and Online Stages

- ❖ MyFitnessPal: Track your day-to-day food consumption, put forth wellness objectives, and access a data set of more than 11 million food varieties.
- ❖ Nike Preparing Club: Look over various exercises driven by Nike Expert Coaches, going from strength preparation to yoga and cardio.
- ❖ Headspace: Practice care and reflection with directed meetings intended to decrease pressure and work on general prosperity.

3. Books and Cookbooks

- "The Whole30: The 30-Day Manual for Complete Wellbeing and Food Opportunity" by Melissa Hartwig Metropolitan and Dallas Hartwig: A far-reaching manual for resetting your dietary patterns and working on by and large well-being in 30 days.
- "Eat to Live: The Astounding Supplement Rich Program for Quick and Supported Weight Reduction" by Joel Fuhrman, M.D.: Find out about the wholesome science behind plant-based eating and its advantages for long haul wellbeing.

4. Support Gatherings and Online People Group

- ✓ Reddit: Join well-being-centered subreddits like r/nourishment, r/wellness, or r/loseit to share encounters, get clarification on pressing issues, and track down inspiration from a strong local area.
- ✓ Facebook Groups: Investigate bunches devoted to smart dieting, wellness difficulties, and weight reduction ventures. Associate with peers, share progress, and get support en route.